Toxin-Antitoxin Systems in *Pseudomonas aeruginosa*

Edited by

Mina Mahmoudi
Department of Microbiology
Faculty of Medicine
Ilam University of Medical Sciences
Iran

Sobhan Ghafourian
Department of Microbiology
Faculty of Medicine
Ilam University of Medical Sciences
Iran

&

Behzad Badakhsh
Department of Gastroenterology
Faculty of Medicine
Ilam University of Medical Sciences
Iran

Toxin-Antitoxin Systems in *Pseudomonas aeruginosa*

Editors: Mina Mahmoudi, Sobhan, Ghafourian and Behzad Badakhsh

ISBN (Online): 978-1-68108-793-1

ISBN (Print): 978-1-68108-794-8

ISBN (Paperback): 978-1-68108-795-5

Published by Bentham Science Publishers – Sharjah, UAE. All Rights Reserved.

need for a court order if at any point you breach any terms of this License Agreement. In no event will any delay or failure by Bentham Science Publishers in enforcing your compliance with this License Agreement constitute a waiver of any of its rights.

3. You acknowledge that you have read this License Agreement, and agree to be bound by its terms and conditions. To the extent that any other terms and conditions presented on any website of Bentham Science Publishers conflict with, or are inconsistent with, the terms and conditions set out in this License Agreement, you acknowledge that the terms and conditions set out in this License Agreement shall prevail.

Bentham Science Publishers Ltd.
Executive Suite Y - 2
PO Box 7917, Saif Zone
Sharjah, U.A.E.
Email: subscriptions@benthamscience.net

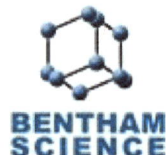

**BENTHAM
SCIENCE**

CONTENTS

FOREWORD

Given the gap in the comprehensive book on *Pseudomonas aeruginosa* and the new findings, the authors decided to address as many important issues as possible about this bacterium. This book is also unique in novel information of *P. aeruginosa*. Still another factor is given by many interesting chapters in detail and plenty of colorful illustrations have been shown. After reading this book, it is hoped that the reader will acquire the necessary knowledge needed for treating patients and promoting useful research designs in eradicating bacteria. By knowing the pathogenesis pathways and new systems in this bacterium, a new horizon will be created in the reader's mind about this bacterium. Writing the book took about two years, with the help of prominent professors and researchers of Ilam University of Medical Sciences, who have been named in different chapters. The authors recommend reading this book to researchers and readers who are looking to solve medical problems in hospitals caused by this bacterium. It is hoped that reading this book will add useful information to readers. In my opinion, the authors would be pleased of having grateful readers who gain broad knowledge for their current practice in Microbiology and Infectious Disease and it will also provide help for their future research.

Mohammad Mehdi Feizabadi
Department of Microbiology
Faculty of Medicine
Tehran University of Medical Science
Tehran
Iran

PREFACE

No one knows exactly when humans and pathogenic bacteria were encountered with each other. But since then, the war began over life and survival between them. During this time, both sides of the war tried to equip themselves with all their might. Throughout time, sometimes humans and sometimes pathogenic bacteria have been victorious, but the contention has not ended yet. However, some of these pathogenic bacteria are stubborn fighters and require much more attention and unfortunately, humans have been disarmed against some of them. Among them, *Pseudomonas aeruginosa* is the pathogen that poses a serious threat to human health. The spectrum of its pathogenesis is very wide. So, the infection can range from a simple superficial infection to a deadly infection. Regrettably, it is one of the most resistant bacteria on the planet, which makes it one of the most prominent and ruthless bacterial fighters.

The present book deals with *P. aeruginosa* and toxin-antitoxin systems in the novel way. This book is recommended not only for interested students but also for those who are interested in research in this field. Currently, *P. aeruginosa* is one of the most essential topics for researchers due to its high pathogenicity and severe antibiotic resistance. On the other hand, toxin-antitoxin systems are considered as one of the most potentially novel antimicrobial targets. In recent years, several scientists have studied the toxin- antitoxin systems in *P. aeruginosa* and their role in pathogenicity, which have also achieved valuable results. Therefore, we have attempted to acquaint the readers with the *P. aeruginosa* as well as one of its most precious therapeutic potentials. However, studies in this area are very rare and limited, but we have tried to provide comprehensive information to the readers.

The chapters of this book are designed in such a way that even readers who have no knowledge of the subject of this book can get acquainted with it throughout the book. Accordingly, the contents of the book have been categorized in three main parts.

First, *P. aeruginosa* has been introduced in different aspects. In this section, readers will become familiar with this microorganism by studying the structure, pathogenicity, antibiotic resistance, and other features of this bacterium. It allows the readers to have almost complete information about the *P. aeruginosa*. Second, classification, structures and roles of toxin antitoxin systems in pathogenicity are explained, which determines how they are involved in the gene regulation and pathogenicity of the bacteria. Therefore, the reader will understand the importance and necessity of recognizing these systems. Third, well-known toxin-antitoxin systems and their functions have been discussed in *P. aeruginosa*. Indeed, we tried to provide useful information in an explicit way. At the end of the book, we hope that the readers will be almost ready to join other researchers by the approximate dominance to the topic. In addition, we look forward to be able to make a contribution to the advancement of science in this area.

Mina Mahmoudi
Department of Microbiology
Faculty of Medicine
Ilam University of Medical Sciences
Iran

Sobhan Ghafourian
Department of Microbiology
Faculty of Medicine
Ilam University of Medical Sciences
Iran

&

Behzad Badakhsh
Department of Gastroenterology
Faculty of Medicine
Ilam University of Medical Sciences
Iran

ACKNOWLEDGEMENTS

We would like to express our deepest gratitude to God almighty for benefitting us with his kindness and support at all times. He gave us an opportunity to flourish and allowed us to be immersed in his unique molecular world, the blessings that only a few humans have benefited from.

We humbly extend thanks to our families for the patience and kindness that they showed at the time of writing this book.

We would like to express our sincere gratitude to all the individuals who accompanied us on this route.

This book is dedicated to all people who love the world of micromolecule and do not hesitate to know about it.

Mina Mahmoudi
Department of Microbiology
Faculty of Medicine
Ilam University of Medical Sciences
Iran

Sobhan Ghafourian
Department of Microbiology
Faculty of Medicine
Ilam University of Medical Sciences
Iran

&

Behzad Badakhsh
Department of gastroenterology Faculty of Medicine
Ilam University of Medical Sciences
Iran

List of Contributors

Abbas Maleki	Clinical Microbiology Research Center, Ilam University of Medical Sciences, Ilam, Iran
Behzad Badakhsh	Department of Internal Medicine, Ilam University of Medical Sciences, Ilam, Iran
Hossein Kazemian	Department of Microbiology, Faculty of Medicine, Ilam University of Medical Sciences, Ilam, Iran
Mina Mahmoudi	Department of Microbiology, Faculty of Medicine, Ilam University of Medical Sciences, Ilam, Iran
Nasrin Dayjourian (English Editor)	Library and Documentation Expert, Information Technology Department, Hamedan Agricultural and Natural Resources and Education Center, AREEO, Hamedan, Iran
Nourkhoda Sadeghifard	Department of Microbiology, Faculty of Medicine, Ilam University of Medical Sciences, Ilam, Iran
Sobhan Ghafourian	Department of Microbiology, Faculty of Medicine, Ilam University of Medical Sciences, Ilam, Iran
Zahra Ahmadi (English Editor)	Faculty of Literature and Human Science, Payame Noor University, Ilam, Iran

CHAPTER 1

An Overview of *Pseudomonas aeruginosa*

M. Mahmoudi[1], S. Ghafourian[1,*] and B. Badakhsh[2]

[1] Department of Microbiology, Faculty of Medicine, Ilam University of Medical Sciences, Ilam, Iran

[2] Department of Gastroenterology, Faculty of Medicine, Ilam University of Medical Sciences, Ilam, Iran

Abstract: *Pseudomonas aeruginosa* is an absolute aerobic gram-negative bacterium that has attracted the attention of many researchers for many years. There are plenty of reasons to research on *P. aeruginosa* , which unfortunately has made it an invincible bacterium. Adaptation to environmental changes is one of the most important capabilities that organisms need to survive. This rule also applies to the world of bacteria. *P. aeruginosa* is one of the most well-known bacteria in terms of adaptation to a variety of biological environments. Besides, *P. aeruginosa* has a variety of hosts, including humans. It is known as an opportunistic pathogen, therefore infections caused by *P. aeruginosa* are highly important in immunocompromised patients and it is a major cause of mortality and morbidity in cystic fibrosis patients. Also, *P. aeruginosa* is the most important cause of nosocomial infections, which can seriously threaten the lives of hospitalized patients. Severe resistance to most antibiotics is one of the other reasons for its success in causing infection and survival. *P. aeruginosa* can produce many powerful virulent factors that create unique properties in this bacterium. In this chapter, the general characteristics of *P. aeruginosa* are briefly and usefully explained. So, the reader can get a good idea of this bacterium in a short glance.

Keywords: Overview, *Pseudomonas aeruginosa*.

Among all life-threatening bacteria, the name of *Pseudomonas aeruginosa (P. aeruginosa)* is always shining due to its incredible capacity to stay alive and to destroy its hosts. Initially, it is best to have an overview of the general characteristics of *P. aeruginosa* to be much more ready for more interesting content of the present book.

P. aeruginosa is a Gram-negative bacterium [1], which is not only obligate aerobe but can also utilize other alternative electron acceptors such as nitrate and can

---
** **Corresponding author S. Ghafourian:** Department of Microbiology, Faculty of Medicine, Ilam University of Medical Sciences, Iran; E-mail: sobhan.ghafurian@gmail.com*

survive as a facultative anaerobic microorganism at the same time [2, 3]. It is rod-shaped, asprogenous, non-acid-fast and catalase-positive [4].

Besides, *P. aeruginosa* is a monotrichous flagellated bacterium [5], which makes it different from other fluorescent *Pseudomonads* (*P. putida, P. florescent, etc.*) [6], and versatile by one or several polar flagella [7]. Its rod measuring about 0.6 × 2 μm that can be seen as a single bacterium, in pairs and rarely in short chains (pearlescent) [8]. *P. aeruginosa* appears as multiple colony type that can be considered as different bacteria by non-expert individuals [9]. Generally, two kinds of the colony can be recognized on the agar media. Firstly, it appears as a large and smooth colony with a flat edge and an outstanding center called a fried egg. It is usually isolated from clinical sources. Secondly, it looks rough and outstanding, which is related to natural sources. There is another type, which looks mucous and it is usually isolated from respiratory and urinary secretions [10]. However, the colony of *P. aeruginosa* has grape-like or tortilla-like odor due to the production of trimethylamine [11, 12]. The optimal temperature for growth is 25°C to 37°C [13]. Also, one of the different features of *P. aeruginosa* , is its ability to grow at 42°C, which distinguishes it from many other fluorescent *Pseudomonas* species [14]. The genome size of *P. aeruginosa* is approximately 5.5–7 Mbp with 65–67% of G+C content [15]. It is also able to use the general source of carbon and nitrogen [16]. *P. aeruginosa* can use variety of organic molecules, which leads this bacterium to be very ubiquitous [17]. Almost, *P. aeruginosa* can tolerate hard conditions that's why it is widespread in the environments [18], so, it can be found in soil, water (even distilled water), sewage and specifically in the hospital [19, 20]. In addition, this remarkable property allows *P. aeruginosa* to be the pathogen for a wide range of hosts including, animals, plants, and humans [21]. In particular, this is an opportunistic and serious pathogen in abnormal host defense, severe burns and cystic fibrosis patients [6, 22, 23]. Indeed, *P. aeruginosa* is responsible for multiple infections, which can vary from local to systemic as well as the illness severity can be diverse from benign to life-threatening diseases [24].

Many strains of *P. aeruginosa* produce different kinds of pigments that some of them can dissolve in water and diffuse to the media and some of them are associated with the cell mass. The pigments are prominent to use diagnostic purposes due to its special features. For instance, the pyoverdin is a fluorescent pigment of *P. aeruginosa* and appears in a yellow-green color that can be seen in a low concentration of iron. In addition, the pyocyanin is the most famous characteristic pigment with the blue-green color. The color of pyocyanin is pH-dependent and it turns red in acidic environments [15]. The pyosyanin is toxic for the ciliated epithelium of the respiratory tract as well as it has a bactericidal effect on *Escherichia coli* (*E. coli*), *Staphylococcus aureus* (*S. aureus*), *Mycobacterium semegmatis* [22, 23]. The phenazine-α-carboxylate and chlororaphin can also be seen in orange and green, respectively. The pyorubin can be seen in red color.

Eventually, the pyomelanin is a brown color. There are also some other pigments such as oxychlororaphin *etc.* [7].

Finally, it may be possible to highlight the importance of *P. aeruginosa* in a few lines. So, it drives its ability to distribute in the most and hard conditions in nature, having very strong and potent pathogenesis factors and be resistant to most of the antibacterial agents, which makes it one of the most resistant and recalcitrant organisms in the world of creatures.

CONSENT FOR PUBLICATION

Not applicable.

CONFLICT OF INTEREST

The authors declare no conflict of interest, financial or otherwise.

ACKNOWLEDGEMENTS

Declared none.

REFERENCES

[1]   Ramalingam B, Parandhaman T, Das SK. Antibacterial effects of biosynthesized silver nanoparticles on surface ultrastructure and nanomechanical properties of gram-negative bacteria *viz. Escherichia coli* and *Pseudomonas aeruginosa*. ACS Appl Mater Interfaces 2016; 8(7): 4963-76.
[http://dx.doi.org/10.1021/acsami.6b00161] [PMID: 26829373]

[2]   Davies KJ, Lloyd D, Boddy L. The effect of oxygen on denitrification in *Paracoccus denitrificans* and *Pseudomonas aeruginosa*. J Gen Microbiol 1989; 135(9): 2445-51.
[PMID: 2516869]

[3]   Louie TJ, Bartlett JG, Tally FP, Gorbach SL. Aerobic and anaerobic bacteria in diabetic foot ulcers. Ann Intern Med 1976; 85(4): 461-3.
[http://dx.doi.org/10.7326/0003-4819-85-4-461] [PMID: 970773]

[4]   Wu W, Jin Y, Bai F, Jin S. *Pseudomonas aeruginosa*. Molecular Medical Microbiology. Elsevier 2015; pp. 753-67.

[5]   Vaituzis Z, Doetsch RN. Motility tracks: technique for quantitative study of bacterial movement. Appl Microbiol 1969; 17(4): 584-8.
[http://dx.doi.org/10.1128/AM.17.4.584-588.1969] [PMID: 4977222]

[6]   Klockgether J, Tümmler B. Recent advances in understanding *Pseudomonas aeruginosa* as a pathogen. F1000 Res 2017; 6: 1261.
[http://dx.doi.org/10.12688/f1000research.10506.1] [PMID: 28794863]

[7]   Brooks G, Carroll K, Butel J, Morse S, Mietzner T. Adelberg Medical Microbiology: Placebo doo 2015.

[8]   Kirisits MJ, Prost L, Starkey M, Parsek MR. Characterization of colony morphology variants isolated

from *Pseudomonas aeruginosa* biofilms. Appl Environ Microbiol 2005; 71(8): 4809-21.
[http://dx.doi.org/10.1128/AEM.71.8.4809-4821.2005] [PMID: 16085879]

[9]   Todar K. Todar's online textbook of bacteriology 2004.

[10]   Wood CL, Tanner BD, Higgins LA, Dennis JS, Luempert LG III. Effectiveness of a steam cleaning unit for disinfection in a veterinary hospital. Am J Vet Res 2014; 75(12): 1083-8.
[http://dx.doi.org/10.2460/ajvr.75.12.1083] [PMID: 25419808]

[11]   Baron S. Alphaviruses (Togaviridae) and Flaviviruses (Flaviviridae)--Medical Microbiology: University of Texas Medical Branch at Galveston 1996.

[12]   Ng W. Effect of temperature on growth of Pseudomonas protegens Pf-5 and *Pseudomonas aeruginosa* PRD-10 in LB Lennox medium. PeerJ Preprints 2018; 2167-9843.

[13]   Borriello S, Murray P, Funke G. Topley & Wilson's Microbiology & Microbial infections. ASM press 2005.

[14]   Tassios PT, Gennimata V, Maniatis AN, Fock C, Legakis NJ. The Greek *Pseudomonas aeruginosa* Study Group. Emergence of multidrug resistance in ubiquitous and dominant *Pseudomonas aeruginosa* serogroup O:11. J Clin Microbiol 1998; 36(4): 897-901.
[http://dx.doi.org/10.1128/JCM.36.4.897-901.1998] [PMID: 9542905]

[15]   Dinesh SD, Grundmann H, Pitt TL, Römling U. European-wide distribution of *Pseudomonas aeruginosa* clone C. Clin Microbiol Infect 2003; 9(12): 1228-33.
[http://dx.doi.org/10.1111/j.1469-0691.2003.00793.x] [PMID: 14686989]

[16]   Pirnay JP, Matthijs S, Colak H, *et al.* Global *Pseudomonas aeruginosa* biodiversity as reflected in a Belgian river. Environ Microbiol 2005; 7(7): 969-80.
[http://dx.doi.org/10.1111/j.1462-2920.2005.00776.x] [PMID: 15946293]

[17]   Favero MS, Carson LA, Bond WW, Petersen NJ. *Pseudomonas aeruginosa*: growth in distilled water from hospitals. Science 1971; 173(3999): 836-8.
[http://dx.doi.org/10.1126/science.173.3999.836] [PMID: 4999114]

[18]   Mashhady MA, Abkhoo J, Jahani S, Abyar S, Khosravani F. Inhibitory Effects of Plant Extracts on *Pseudomonas aeruginosa* Biofilm Formation. Int J Infect 2016; 3(4): e38199.
[http://dx.doi.org/10.17795/iji.38199]

[19]   Lang AB, Horn MP, Imboden MA, Zuercher AW. Prophylaxis and therapy of *Pseudomonas aeruginosa* infection in cystic fibrosis and immunocompromised patients. Vaccine 2004; 22(Suppl. 1): S44-8.
[http://dx.doi.org/10.1016/j.vaccine.2004.08.016] [PMID: 15576201]

[20]   Lyczak JB, Cannon CL, Pier GB. Establishment of *Pseudomonas aeruginosa* infection: lessons from a versatile opportunist. Microbes Infect 2000; 2(9): 1051-60.
[http://dx.doi.org/10.1016/S1286-4579(00)01259-4] [PMID: 10967285]

[21]   Estahbanati HK, Kashani PP, Ghanaatpisheh F. Frequency of *Pseudomonas aeruginosa* serotypes in burn wound infections and their resistance to antibiotics. Burns 2002; 28(4): 340-8.
[http://dx.doi.org/10.1016/S0305-4179(02)00024-4] [PMID: 12052372]

[22]   Gillespie S, Hawkey PM. Principles and practice of clinical bacteriology. John Wiley & Sons 2006.
[http://dx.doi.org/10.1002/9780470017968]

[23]   Rada B, Leto TL. Pyocyanin effects on respiratory epithelium: relevance in *Pseudomonas aeruginosa* airway infections. Trends Microbiol 2013; 21(2): 73-81.
[http://dx.doi.org/10.1016/j.tim.2012.10.004] [PMID: 23140890]

[24]   Taghinejad J, Hosseinzadeh M, Molayi Kohneshahri S, Javan Jasor V. *Pseudomonas aeruginosa*: A biological review. Laboratory & Diagnosis 2017; 8(34): 67-82.

CHAPTER 2

History and Etymology

M. Mahmoudi[1], S. Ghafourian[1,*], N. Sadeghifard[1] and B. Badakhsh[2]

[1] *Department of Microbiology, Faculty of Medicine, Ilam University of Medical Sciences, Ilam, Iran*

[2] *Department of Gastroenterology, Faculty of Medicine, Ilam University of Medical Sciences, Ilam, Iran*

Abstract: The greenish-blue color dye on the wounds and bandages of patients was the first characteristic that attracted the attention of researchers in the discovery of this bacterium. Eventually, in 1882, a French pharmacist, Carle Gessard discovered *P. aeruginosa* from colored cutaneous wounds. He also suggested that this bacterium may be associated with many diseases. Over time, this bacterium found its special niche in the biological and medical sciences due to the complexity, the production of various extracellular products, and the lack of information on how exactly the disease is caused. Along with these findings, several names were assigned to this bacillus bacterium. Finally, *Pseudomonas aeruginosa* was assigned based on the meaning and concept of title root and appearance of the bacterium. In a general sense, *Pseudomonas aeruginosa* was referred to the identical units of cells that produced a significant amount of greenish-blue color.

Keywords: Discovery, Etymology, History, *P. aeruginosa*.

In the 1850s, someone named Sedillot noticed the greenish-blue color stains on the bandage and clothes of patients and surgeons, whether they can be the cause of severe disease or not. But he didn't succeed in understanding the reason of it.

Ten years later (the 1860s), Ferdos could extract the pigments from the stains as a crystalline substance and named it pyocyanin. After that, Luke explained that the greenish-blue stains are associated with infections and claimed that he has seen rod shape elements in pus in 1862s. Eventually, a pharmacist from Paris, France, Carle Gessard isolated the *P. aeruginosa* from a cutaneous wound, which had greenish-blue color in 1882s. He also discovered that this pigment is water-soluble and illuminate under the ultra-violate light and named it *Bacillus pyocyaneus*. Finally, he concluded that this bacilli bacterium is a pathogen and

---

[*] **Corresponding author S. Ghafourian:** Department of Microbiology, Faculty of Medicine, Ilam University of Medical Sciences, Iran; E-mail: sobhan.ghafurian@gmail.com

probably is associated with lots of diseases. In 1889, Charrin considered the role of *P. aeruginosa* in pathogenesis in animals. Then, Migula explained the rudimentary characterization of *P. aeruginosa* in 1894s. Subsequently, Wasserman showed that the role of toxin and extracellular material is much more prominent than the bacterial mass in 1896s. Ultimately, in 1925s, Olser noticed the role of *P. aeruginosa* to the secondary infectious. With the passage of time, the importance of *P. aeruginosa* becomes more highlighted and as of now, it is one of the main factors of nosocomial infections. Over time, this bacilli bacterium allocated several names based on its features. Here, we just give a brief note of them, which are as follows: *Bacterium aeruginosom, Bacterium aeruginosum, Micrococcus pyocyaneus, Bacillus aeruginosus, Bacillus pyocyaneus, Pseudomonas pyocyanea, Bacterium pyocyaneum, and Pseudomonas polycolor.*

Finally, *P. aeruginosa* was assigned as a final name. However, how this name was chosen is associated with the root and etymology of the title of *Pseudomonas aeruginosa* [1, 2].

The German botanist, Walter Migula observed and explained a genus, as "Cells with polar organs of motility" and allocated the term *Pseudomonas* for them in 1894.

The *pseudo* ("false") + *monas* ("unit") is originated from Greek. In addition, in 1773 a Danish naturist Otto Friedrich Müller invented the term *Monas* to explain ciliate protozoans genus means "infusoria". He described this organism as a tiny, simple, transparent and worm-like microorganism.

Therefore, There is another theory which states that Walter Migula did not select Greek words directly. Indeed, probably he used *Monas* ("unit") to explain those cells, which had a similar relative extent and active mobility.

Generally, *Pseudomonas aeruginosa* has been taken from the Latin language, so, it is an adjective and feminine of aerūginōsus term. The aerūgō means verdigris that can be related to the green color of copper rust as well as −ōsus added to the aerūgō to create an adjective indicating redundancy and intensity of aerūgō as a noun. By taking a glance at *Pseudomonas aeruginosa* term, it can be simply referring to the similar units of cells, which produce a great measure of greenish-blue color [3 - 5].

CONSENT FOR PUBLICATION

Not applicable.

CONFLICT OF INTEREST

The authors declare no conflict of interest, financial or otherwise.

ACKNOWLEDGEMENTS

Declared none.

REFERENCES

[1]   Buchanan R, Buchanan R, Gibbons N. Bergey's Manual of Determinative Bacteriology. William's and Wilkins Company 1970.

[2]   Gransden WR. Topley and Wilson's Microbiology and Microbial Infections. J Clin Pathol 9th edition(CD-ROM).. 1999; 52(3): 237-8.

[3]   Etymologia: Pseudomonas. Emerg Infect Dis 2012; 18(8): 1241. [http://dx.doi.org/10.3201/eid1808.ET1808]

[4]   Dorland NW. Dorland's illustrated medical dictionary. 32nd., Elsevier/Saunders Philadelphia 2012.

[5]   Palleroni NJ. The pseudomonas story. Environ Microbiol 2010; 12(6): 1377-83. [http://dx.doi.org/10.1111/j.1462-2920.2009.02041.x] [PMID: 20553550]

CHAPTER 3

Virulence Factors of *P. aeruginosa* and Their Role in Pathogenicity

M. Mahmoudi[1], S. Ghafourian[1,*], A. Maleki[2] and B. Badakhsh[3]

[1] *Department of Microbiology, Faculty of Medicine, Ilam University of Medical Sciences, Ilam, Iran*

[2] *Clinical Microbiology Research Center, Ilam University of Medical Sciences, Ilam, Iran*

[3] *Department of Gastroenterology, Faculty of Medicine, Ilam University of Medical Sciences, Ilam, Iran*

Abstract: *P. aeruginosa* can cause a variety of infections in different hosts. For this purpose, it regulates several virulence factors depending on the surrounding conditions and environments. As a result, the type and severity of diseases vary from host to host. For instance, it causes acute infection in some patients, while it causes chronic infections in others. On the other hand, it can sometimes be very deadly and sometimes easy to treat. The difference in the behavior of *P. aeruginosa* is directly related to the expression of key virulence factors. In this chapter, major virulence factors and their roles in pathogenicity that are related to human diseases are comprehensively discussed. These virulence factors including, lipopolysaccharide, adhesions, lectins, alginate, flagella, pigments, biofilm, toxins, enzymes, proteases, *etc*. It should be noted that recognition and familiarity with virulence factors can be very helpful and effective to understand *P. aeruginosa* pathogenesis. Therefore, we discussed the structure as well as the manner of virulence factors intervention in *P. aeruginosa* infections. We hope to create a general idea of *P. aeruginosa* structure in the minds of the readers at the end of this chapter.

Keywords: Pathogenicity, Structure, Virulence factor.

As was mentioned earlier, *P. aeruginosa* is associated with a variety of acute and chronic infections that can happen in immunocompromised and the other patients. Some studies demonstrated that *P. aeruginosa* is responsible for several fatal diseases, which can occur even in patients with a normal immune system. Accordingly, the ability of *P. aeruginosa* to create a wide spectrum of diseases must be associated with many virulence factors [1]. However, not all of the virulence factors are available in all isolates. Obviously, the up-regulation and

* **Corresponding author S. Ghafourian:** Department of Microbiology, Faculty of Medicine, Ilam University of Medical Sciences, Iran; E-mail:sobhan.ghafurian@gmail.com

Mina Mahmoudi, Sobhan Ghafourian & Behzad Badakhsh (Eds.)

down-regulation of the virulence factors create different types of isolates. For more clarity , the chronic infection isolates are different in terms of phenotypic features by acute infection isolates [2]. Actually, the acute infection isolates express a lot of virulence factors compare with chronic infection isolates. For instance, during the lung chronic infection in cystic fibrosis (CF) patients, some of the most important virulence factors, which are involved in inflammation, are down-regulated or the lack of them has severely occurred. In detail, during the early (acute) lung infection in CF patients, the majority of toxins and enzymes are secreted [3]. The Lipopolysaccharides (LPS) that are one of the causes of fever in the acute infection are in complete mode. The wild type LPS contains an O-antigen chain, so-called smooth LPS(sLPS) can stimulate the immune system strongly. In addition, the flagella, type IV pili expressed nicely, and a low level of alginate are available in acute lung infection in CF patients.

In contrast, the secretion of virulence factors is decreased in a chronic infection that happens due to the adaption of *P. aeruginosa* with the lung environments. More precisely, the LPS structure does not contain the O-antigen chain and terms as rough LPS(rLPS). Actually, this is a defective form of LPS. In addition, the lipid A will be deacylated. Despite the auxotrophy can be seen in this mode, some other components such as alginate, suffer with the increasing of their overexpression level. *P. aeruginosa* isolates that are attended to chronic infection are more readily to form biofilm or construct mucoid mass [4].

Generally, the effect of *P. aeruginosa* virulence factors can facilitate adhesion and then disrupt the host cell signaling [5]. Hence, they have such putative virulence factors that in some cases cause their host to die.

Therefore, different conditions and environments are involved in the regulation of *P.aeruginosa* virulence factor genes. In the following, we describe the virulence factors of *P. aeruginosa* briefly for further illustrating the structure and potential of its pathogenicity.

1. LIPOPOLYSACCHARIDE (LPS)

Perhaps, the LPS could be considered as the most prominent component of the outer membrane or the key virulence factor of *P. aeruginosa* [6]. The LPS is the common outer leaflet of Gram-negative outer membrane bacteria [4]. The most significant issue about the LPS is its role in the pathogenesis of the bacteria. Therefore, this is physical barrier, which can protect the bacteria from host defense [6]. It is referred as endotoxin and interacts with the host cells as well as antibiotic molecules. The LPS can trigger cell signaling that can lead to cell disruption and bacteremia [7].

Generally, the LPS molecule has three domains that consist of lipid A, core and O-antigen. The lipid A is a hydrophobic domain and it is responsible for the endotoxicity feature of the LPS. Also, the core is a non-repeating oligosaccharide and the O-antigen is the distal polysaccharide [8].

In *P. aeruginosa*, lipid A is the basic domain, which has a disaccharide backbone containing N- and O-acylated diglucosamine bisphosphate backbone [4-P-β-D-GlcpNII-(1→6)-α-D-GlcpNI-(1→P] that attached to many fatty acid molecules, which leads to the anchor of LPS to the inner membrane. In some cases, the chemical alternation can be happening in the number of primary acyl groups and type of fatty acids. Hence, they will be replaced with primary and secondary acyl groups. The variation in the amount of accessible magnesium is one of the effective reasons for the pattern of acylation in lipid A molecule [6].

In all wild type isolates of *P. aeruginosa*, lipid A is attached to approximately ten branched oligosaccharides, which named core domain. In addition, the preponderance of fatty acids in lipid A structure is directly associated with the potency of the pathogenicity.

The second domain of LPS is a core that is located next to and after lipid A.

In Gram-negative bacteria, the core domain is divided into two parts including outer core and inner core. The inner core consists of heptose phosphate, ethanolamine heptose phosphate and 2-keto-3-deoxy-octonate (KDO) that is attached to lipidA (α2→6) by the acid susceptible ketosidic bond. The phosphate and KDO have a negative charge and bind to the divalent metal cations. Then, they cause outer membrane stabilization and an obstacle to hydrophobic molecules. The permeability of the cell membrane depends on these cations. For instance, the Ethylenediaminetetraacetic acid (EDTA) as a chelating agent of cations as well as polycationic antibiotics such as polymyxin and aminoglycosides are leading to the permeability of the great hydrophobic molecules.

Subsequently, the outer core consists of glucose, galactose, and N-acetylglucosamine [9]. Eventually, the last domain of the LPS is an O-antigen. It consists of repeated polymeric carbohydrate that attached to the core by the covalent bonds [10].

There are two types of O-antigen in terms of their structure and serological features in *P. aeruginosa*. This difference is based on their biosynthesis mechanism and they are named A-band (common) and B-band (O-specific). The A-band is a homopolymer of D-rhamnose and it is approximately 70 sugars long. The B-band has more importance due to its ability to trigger severe immune response compare with A-band. Due to this property of B-band, it is used for serotyping of *P. aeruginosa* isolates. At present, there are 20 serotypes of *P. aeruginosa* based on their O-antigen composition. Structurally, the B-band is heteropolymer and it is different among the strains in terms of chain length and nature of the sugar.

Remarkably, some of the strains are not able to produce any O-polysaccharide and it leads to create rough colonies. Also, some of them have only one O-saccharide that forms semi-rough colonies. Finally, those isolates, which have an O-antigen side chain, constitute smooth colonies [1].

In particular, the sublime importance of LPS is its ability to activate innate immunity (TLR4, NLRP1, NLRP2, and NLRP3) and also acquired immunity. The recognition of the LPS usually happens by the macrophage and dendritic cells *etc.* The LPS bond to the TLR4–MD2–CD14 complex of immune cells, but the lipid A needs another protein to be identified means LPS-binding protein (LBP) that converts oligomeric micelles of LPS binds to the monomer in order to deliver to CD14 molecule. On the other hand, the NLRs lead to the pyroptosis, inflammation, and production of the inflammasome [8].Although the LPS generates great amounts of immune response but LPS derived vaccines have not been successful yet [11].

2. ADHESIONS

2.1. Type IV Pili (TFP)

TFP is a unique weapon that not only plays a crucial role just in the pathogenesis of *P. aeruginosa* but also in some other bacteria including, *N. gonorrhoeae, N. meningitidis, M. bovis, E. corrodens, V. cholerae, EPEC,* and enterotoxigenic *E. coli.*The role of the TFP is very predominant in pathogenesis, so strains lacking type IV pili are not infectious [9]. Generally, the TFP involves normal motility, twitching, adhesion, virulence, biofilm formation and cell-cell aggregation [12 - 14]. In terms of structure, it is long and thin so that it has a 5-8 nm diameter [15]. When the TFP is contacted by a receptor at the surface, signals are generated inside the bacteria. On one hand, the TFP acts as a mechanical sensor, especially when the *P. aeruginosa* contacts with the solid surfaces. On the other hand, the Chp system, which consists of two subunits, regulates the expression of the TFP. Some studies claimed that, when the Chp protein does not exist, the assembly of the TFP and subsequently, the twitching motility would be disrupted [16]. From a general perspective, the planktonic *P. aeruginosa* swims within liquid space with the aid of flagella [17]. Here, if the TFP contacts with its target cells, it will be modified, which is not completely understood. Then, two chemosensory proteins, pilJ and PilA transduce the signal inside of the bacterial cell. By the generation of this interior signal, the cAMP also produced. The cAMP is one of the varieties of the signaling molecules and binds to the Vfr (virulence factor regulator). Finally, the Vfr stimulates the transcription of genes that are more than 100. For instance, the Vfr activates type II and III secretion systems, which are very important in the first stage of pathogenicity and this leads to the starting of the acute phase of the disease [18]. On the other hand, Vfr also activates the quorum sensing system that will stimulate the production of autoinducers [19].

As was mentioned, the TFP also participates in biofilm formation. The biofilm is a unique structure that causes antimicrobial resistance, persistent and chronic infections [20]. TFP is the structural component in the matrix of biofilm. In the early stages of biofilm formation, TFP plays a role in adherence to the surfaces and then it interferes in formation of the microcolonies [21].

Another role that has been defined for TFP is a phage receptor for DLP1 and DLP2 bacteriophages [22]. In addition, by the loss of fibronectin by proteases in epithelial cells, TFP receptors, asialo-GM1 and asialo-GM2 will be available for the *P. aeruginosa*. Therefore, using the receptors of these damaged cells; trachea infection will begin [23]. All of these capabilities point to the importance of this particular type of pili in infectious and pathogenesis.

2.2. Lectins

There are two major lectins of *P. aeruginosa*, LecA, and LecB. They are also named as PA-IL and PA-IIL and they have 12.8 kDa and 11.9 kDa weight, respectively [24 - 27]. Both lecA and lecB play several roles such as, adhesion of the bacteria to the host cells or each other, which leads to tissue damage and participates in biofilm formation. To perform mentioned actions, lecA and lecB must interact with their specific receptors at the surfaces of interest (such as epithelial cells). Hence, the lecA binds to the D-galactose or N-acetyl-D-galactosamine and the lecB binds to the L-fucose or mannose [26].

As it is obvious, one of the most important stages of pathogenicity is adhesion. Successful adhesion of bacteria to the desired surface leads to colonization, invasion or in some cases formation of the biofilm. For the adhesion purpose, there are a lot of both lectins, which are located on the surface of *P. aeruginosa* [25, 28]. Other roles are considered for these two lectins, which in some cases are indirectly related to adhesion. However, separately, the lecA causes respiratory epithelial injury as well as effects on the penetration of the intestinal epithelium that leads to the high absorption of other virulence factors such as exotoxin A [29]. On the other hand, the lecB also participates the activity of protease IV and biogenesis of pilus [30, 31].

2.3. Alginate

Alginate linear polymer molecules demonstrated a variety of effects on properties of bacterial surface including, charge, hydrophobicity and cell-surface electrostatic interaction with the surface [32]. Structurally, it consists of (1~4)-linked exopolysaccharide of β-D-mannuronic acid and C-5 epimer α-L-guluronic [33]. In addition, a species of brown seaweeds also can produce alginate, which is called *Phaeophyceae* [34]. However, not all the bacteria can produce alginate, but a few species such as *P. aeruginosa*, *P. fluorescens,* and *P. syringae* are defined as alginate producer bacteria [33, 35, 36], while many genes are involved in synthesis of alginate (*AlgD* is the main), which is encoded by most important regulatory enzyme, GDP-mannose dehydrogenase [37]. The keys regulators for the synthesis of the alginate are KCl and NaCl, which cause activation of *algD* promoter. Hence, the lungs of Cystic Fibrosis patients are an ideal site for activation of the alginate due to the high concentration of Na^+, Cl^-, Ca^{2+} and K^+ [38].

The alginate plays a role as a capsular polysaccharide in the formation of the biofilm, so it is one of the main components in the construction of the extracellular polysaccharide matrix of the biofilm [39].

Based on the previews study, alginate causes over activation of the immune response in CF patients, which leads to tissue damage in the lungs [40]. Since the role of alginate in biofilm formation has been proven, it can also be one of the factors for the creation of persistency even under the antibiotic therapy condition [41]. On the other hand, it is also hydrophiles the surface of the bacterial cells and inhibits phagocytosis [42].

2.4. Flagella

Motility is considered as the most significant role of flagella among bacteria, which can also definitely extend to *P. aeruginosa* [43]. It may seem that motility does not have a clear role in the development of the disease but it should be noted that the motility plays a key role in the creation of various mechanisms and features in *P. aeruginosa*. Besides, although the role of the pili in adhesion is prominent, there are new studies, which have suggested flagella as adhesion organ, too [44, 45]. There is a specific protein inside the structure of *P. aeruginosa* flagella, FliD, which is responsible for the adhesion to respiratory mucins [46]. However, the corneal cells are the other example of the adhesion site of the flagella. Another role assigned to the flagella is the creation of the invasion. Therefore, mutants are less invasive in comparison to the strains [43]. The flagella also involved in the inflammatory response of the host. The toll-like-receptor 5(TLR5) is the mediator for all bacterial flagella not only for *P. aeruginosa* but the specific binding site for *P. aeruginosa* flagella is leucine-rich repeat region part of TLR5. Eventually, chemotaxis that helps the bacteria to gain nutrients also appertains to the flagella to swim [47, 48].

3. PIGMENTS

Perhaps, *P. aeruginosa* can be considered as the most beautiful and eye-catching bacteria in the world of microorganisms. This amazing property is due to its ability to produce several types of pigments. Hitherto, many pigments are discovered in *P. aeruginosa*, which we will explain most important of them below.

3.1. Pyoverdine

Pyoverdine or Psudobactin is one of the important pigments of *P. aeruginosa* , which produces yellow-green color. The association between production of pyoverdine and iron uptake has been proven properly. Hence, when there is a limitation of iron in the environment, pyoverdine transports iron and so-called siderophore [49]. This issue demonstrates that pyoverdine can be very helpful for successful colonization under the limitation of nutrients. So, with attention to its high importance in the survival of bacteria, there are two groups of *Pseudomonas* species based on the production of pyoverdine. Given that pyoverdine pigments have fluorescent properties, the first group is called fluorescent group including, *P. aeruginosa, P. chlororaphis, P. fluorescens, P. monteilii, P. putida, P. plecoglossidica, P. simiae, P. syringae*. The second group is also named non-fluorescent group including, *P. alcaligenes, P. anguilliseptica, P. fragi, P. mendocina, P. stutzeri, P. pseudoalcaligenes* [50].

The function of pyoverdine and the iron absorption by it is the most predominant issue about this pigment. Therefore, we will briefly describe it in the following. After the biosynthesis of the pyoverdine inside the cytoplasm, it will go to the environment by the efflux pumps to sequester iron. After the acquisition of iron, it must be back to the bacteria. For this purpose, there is specific outer membrane transporter, which is called FvpA. In addition, the receptor of the FvpA is TonB, which is the energy-transducing protein. On the other hand, there is the TonB-ExbB-ExbD complex, which is located inside the inner membrane and contains the tonB box. The FvpA configuration will change by the receiving iron complex, which leads to interaction between TonB and TonB box. Eventually, the ferric siderophore transports inside the cell [51].

The gaining of iron is a vital issue for bacteria, so, there is a silent war and huge competition for obtaining the iron. It is because of the participation of iron in cellular processes such as replication of DNA, generation of energy, transportation of oxygen, *etc.* Accordingly, pathogens that are equipped to obtain iron have a better chance of survival [52].

3.2. Pyocyanin

Pyocyanin belongs to the phenazine group that consists of nitrogen-containing heterocyclic compounds. This is the color-dependent pigment. So, the blue-greenish color can be seen in the neutral pH and in contrast, it becomes red under the acidic condition [53]. It is suggested that pyocyanin is associated with the pathogenicity of the *P. aeruginosa* and is secreted to the environment by the type II secretion system [54]. Hence, it is associated with several kinds of infections and cellular effects that it is explained to them briefly. Accordingly, several studies demonstrated the inflammatory effect of the pyocyanin *in vitro* conditions [54 - 56]. Some other studies have implicated the effect of pyocyanin on the respiratory system. Based on this, pyocyanin causes ciliary dyskinesia, ciliary stasis, and epithelial cell disruption in the respiratory system [57]. Subsequently, *P. aeruginosa* is one of urinary tract infection pathogens, which is mostly isolated from patients with a history of using catheters.

Based on this, there is a study, which showed that the pyocyanin can reduce RT4 urothelial cell viability [58]. In addition, pyocyanin also affects the central nervous system (CNS). Although nervous infections caused by *P. aeruginosa* rarely occurred and it can lead to patients' death. It was observed that all of the pathogenicity factors, which are expressed in this type of disease, have high importance in research areas. Studies on astrocytoma cells have shown that, pyocyanin is associated with the production of acidic vesicular organelles that is the hallmark of autophagy [59]. Accordingly, it was reported that cystic fibrosis patients suffer from endothelial dysfunction [60]. Many other roles have been defined for pyocyanin in pathogenicity including, changing the morphology of the hepatic system [61], and causing diabetes by the prevention of aconitase that is one of the components of Krebs cycle and finally leads to the conduction of diabetes [62, 63].

3.3. Pyorubin

Pyorubin is another phenazine pigment of the *P. aeruginosa*, which can produce rarely reddish pigments [64]. As it is obvious, during the oxidative stress, reactive oxygen intermediates are produced and this leads to the disruption of proteins,

DNA and cells [65]. The bacterial cells follow the same rule and they must deal with oxidative stress to stay alive. Hence, it is believed that pyorubin has protective effects against oxidative stress [64]. On the other hand, the pyorubin also has antibacterial activity, which can help *P. aeruginosa* to be the dominant pathogen of its host [64]. Although, pyorubin is not the only red color producer pigment of *P. aeruginosa*, the emergence of red color in the culture of clinical strains is very low. Nevertheless, the presence of red color in the culture medium can greatly be helpful for the detection of *P. aeruginosa* strains [66].

3.4. Pyomelanin

Reddish-brownish color production in the culture medium can be one of the features of *P. aeruginosa* [67]. Pyomelanin pigment can be the reason for this event that is produced by the catabolism of tyrosine or phenylalanine. Pyomelanin had various functions that can be mentioned as, ultraviolet light protection, energy transduction, defense against oxidative stress, *etc* [68]. Since the reddish-brownish color of *P. aeruginosa* is usually isolated from the lungs of cystic fibrosis patients, a relationship should exist between cystic fibrosis and pyomelanin. Based on this theory, some researchers claimed that, due to the production of pyomelanin, the effect of oxidative stress decreases during the infection by reddish-brownish *P. aeruginosa* isolates in cystic fibrosis patients. Accordingly, pyomelanin pigment has an effective role in the survival of *P. aeruginosa* and the development of chronic infection [69]. In addition, the pyomelanin is also isolated from sputum, urine, and wound samples but as was mentioned the higher amount of isolation of pyomelanin belongs to cystic fibrosis patients.

3.5. Other Pigments

Except for pyocyanin, two other pigments belong to the phenazine group, chlororaphin, and oxychlororaphin. Chlororaphin can be seen in green and oxychlororaphin can be seen in orange. The chlororaphin forms green crystals in the agar media and it is not water-soluble [70]. In contrast, oxychlororaphin is water-soluble [71]. Besides, the phenazine 1-carboxylate is the next pigment of the *P. aeruginosa* that is responsible for the orange color in the culture media. Many studies demonstrated the antibacterial effect of phenazine 1-carboxylate. Therefore, it has been proven that phenazine a-carboxylic acid has a bactericidal effect against *Staphylococcus aureus,* as well as, it can inhibit the growth of *Mycobacterium avium* and *Bacillus anthracis*. The final pigment of the *P. Aeruginosa* names aeruginosa A, which can make the cultured red [72]. It should be noted that the production of the pigments depends on several factors including, available nutrients, exposure to light, pH changes, *etc.* Also in some cases, pigments can be covered by each other and are not always visible.

4. *P. AERUGINOSA* FORMS IN NATURE (PLANKTONIC AND BIOFILM)

Generally, bacteria can be seen in two forms in nature and each of them has different properties and particular symptoms. The first is a planktonic form that can enable the bacteria to move freely in the environment and mostly be independent of others.The planktonic form is responsible for the acute infections that are almost controlled. Although vaccination and antibiotic therapy have been approximately effective in surveillance of acute diseases but with the increase of antibiotic resistance and insufficient render of new antibacterial targets, patients sometimes died. The second form, which is highly important, is a biofilm. The biofilm formation leads to chronic infections such as chronic wounds and otitis media, catheter-associated infections and pneumonia in cystic fibrosis patients. One of the most important issues about biofilm formation is increasing in antibiotic resistance that can lead to significant multiplier resistance [72]. Unfortunately, biofilm formation was identified in 65–80% of all microbial infections [73]. Therefore, fighting against biofilm is one of the main priorities of the field of bacteriology. One of the reasons for researchers' failure to struggle against biofilm is its intricate structure and the complex forming stages.

Therefore, in order to better understanding, we will explain the structure and the procedure of biofilm formation.

Universally, biofilm is an enclosed structure that attaches a population of bacteria to an appropriate surface and protects them against environmental stresses. Some researchers refer to it as the "city of microbes" and subsequently, extracellular polymeric substances (EPS) are "house of the biofilm cells" [74]. The EPS embraces the most crucial and instantaneous bacterial life requirements. That is why there are a variety of components inside the EPS including, extracellular DNA (eDNA), polypeptides, and exopolysaccharides. In the case of *P. aeruginosa* in biofilm stability, three exopolysaccharides are involved, alginate, Pel, and Psl [21].

The role of alginate is more highlighted than the rest. Therefore, alginate protects the biofilm against external harmful agents and maintains water and nutrients [75]. Pel is rich in glucose that is essential for the survival of *P. aeruginosa* [76]. Moreover, eDNA also plays a crucial role in the durability of biofilm. For instance, if the bacteria become famished, the eDNA is available as a nutrient source. On the other hand, eDNA can adhere to bacterial cells to each other and spread the mass of biofilm [77]. In addition, there are other components of the *P. aeruginosa*, which participate in adhesion between materials and biofilm formation including, flagella, type IV pili, *etc.*

As the planktonic *P. aeruginosa* swim inside the liquid environment freely, they could be adhering to the suitable surface *via* irreversible attachment. Then, the EPS matrix produces by them and cells aggregate with each other, which leads to the formation of microcolonies. This structure expands more in this way and biofilms gradually become mature. In the following, the biofilm goes on until it almost covers the desired surface. When the biofilm comes in three-dimensional (3D) form, bacteria, which are enclosed inside it, become protected against antibiotics and other environmental stress extraordinarily. So, bacterial survival increases highly as a consequence.

At this time, planktonic bacteria can egress from the stem of biofilm and go for the new sites of colonization [21]. Based on this, the biofilm formation is defined as an endless cycle and causes chronic infections [78].

We continue the discussion on gene regulation in biofilm formation to better understanding this invincible structure. Several mechanisms and systems are involved in the biofilm formation that we will explain the most important and crucial of them.

The quorum sensing (QS) system, as a modulator for EPS production, has a significant role in biofilm formation [79]. For more information, while the bacterial population density changes in the environment, many genes will be regulated, that called the QS system. In a simple word, bacteria can share information about their density by the autoinducer molecules and subsequently specific genes will be regulated [80]. It seems that QS systems involve in the adaptation of motility, virulence factors, and biofilm formation [81, 82].

Hence, las and rhl are two principal QS systems of the *P. aeruginosa* that are controlling autoinducer molecules N-(3-oxododecanoyl)-L-homoserine lactone (3-oxo-C12-HSL) and N-butanoyl-L-homoserine lactone (C4-HSL). The production of these two autoinducers is under the control of LasI and RhlI. In addition, those two autoinducer are sensed by two transcription factors LasR and RhlR. However, there is another QS system in *P. aeruginosa* named PQS that is associated with acyl-homoserine lactones (AHLs) systems [81]. Moreover, the *psl* operon also is under the regulation by the lasR, which shows the association between QS and production of the psl, main exopolysaccharides of the biofilm matrix [83]. On the other hand, rhl system has been reported as a regulator for the swarming motility that is effective in moving inside the liquid. In addition, another kind of movement is seen in the *P. aeruginosa* that is participated in adherence to surfaces called twitching motility. This movement is provided by the type IV pili [84]. Furthermore, twitching motility is also under the control of QS, which demonstrated the role of IV pili in biofilm formation. Several other factors are under the supervision of QS system such as lectins and rhamnolipids. Based on this, rhl regulates the expression of lecA, lecB and, rhamnolipids [27]. Besides, various functions are defined for the rhamnolipids such as, simplification of microcolonies and 3D structure formation, the release of a planktonic bacterium from a biofilm stem, and creating open channels in biofilm in order to prevent bacterial colonization [85].

As was mentioned before, the biofilm of the *P. aeruginosa* has other regulators, GacS/GacA and RetS/LadS Two-Component Systems [86].While environmental factors stimulate the bacteria, it is sensing and also responding by the two components systems *via* changing the regulation of the genes [87]. Although there are many two-component systems involved in *P. aeruginosa*, the GacS/GacA is one of the most vital of them and can be found in many Gammaproteobacteria, such as *P. aeruginosa*. The importance of this system is due to its ability to regulate a variety of genes, including virulence factors and biofilm formation and quorum sensing [88]. By stimulating GacS, it will be autophosphorylated and the phosphate group will be transferred to the GacA regulator. Subsequently, the GacA up-regulates the expression of RsmZ and RsmY. In this level, there is a small RNA that bounds to the protein RsmA. RsmA is the regulator for the *psl* gene. RsmZ and RsmY inhibit the bounding of the small RNA to RsmA. Therefore, by repressing the RsmA, the *psl* gene will be transcribed and assists in biofilm formation [21]. The next two-component systems are RetS/LadS. The first component, RetS is repressor of the biofilm and in contrast, ladS plays the opposite role, which has histidine kinase activity [89, 90]. It was reported that both the GacS/GacA and RetS/LadS contribute to changing acute to chronic infection [91]. On the other hand, bis-(3'-5')-cyclic dimeric guanosine monophosphate (c-di-GMP) is also playing an important role in biofilm formation by contribution in the production of polysaccharides [92]. Although these molecules are highly found in the bacterial cells, it is suggested that they have a crucial role in many physiological pathways [93] one of them is biofilm formation, so, by increasing the level of c-di-GMP, the production of vital polysaccharides such as alginate and pel will also increase [92]. As was mentioned, these two polysaccharides are the main sugars of biofilm structure, as a result, the high level of c-di-GMP increases biofilm formation [94]. In contrast, it is suggested that by decreasing the level of c-di-GMP, the bacterial motility will be increased *via* the production of flagella [92].

5. TOXINS

5.1. Exotoxin A

Pseudomonas Exotoxin A (PE) is the most prominent virulence factor in *P. aeruginosa*, which generally causes inhibition of protein synthesis, suppression of immune system, direct cythopatic effect, skin necrosis during the burned wound, cornea damage and tissue damage in Chronic Pulmonary Infection. The molecular weight of PE protein is about 5×10^4 dalton with a length of 613 amino acids (aa) [95, 96]. The PE gene translates to the protein by the moncisteronic mRNA [97]. Universally, it is one of the members of the two-component AB toxin family and consists of two main subunits. The A subunit has enzymatic activity and B subunit can bind to the host cells in order to enter the A domain into the cells. In addition, The X-ray crystallography (XRC) technique demonstrated three-dimensional structure of the PE protein that consists of three functional domains [98]. Partially, domains are located as follows from N-terminus to C-terminus direction. The hydrophobic leader peptide with 25 a alengths is standing at the first of the queue and it will be eliminated during the secretion. The receptors binding domain Ia located after the leader peptide. It contains amino acids 1 to 252 and is made from antiparallel beta-sheets. Following them, there is domain II from aa 253 to 364 in the PE protein, which consists of six α-helices and causes the toxin to pass through the membrane. Other residues of domain Ib (aa 365-404) means aa 400 to 404, and domain family, and also domain III that includes aa 405 to 613 creates the catalytic subunit [99]. Moreover, the catalytic subunit belongs to mono-ADP-ribosyltransferase family that determined as a as NAD^+ -diphthamide-ADP-ribosyltransferase enzyme [100].

Even though the expression of the PE protein is not completely clear yet, but it is obvious that it leads to the intoxication of the host cells. On the one hand, the iron ion is one of the most important colonization requirements and several studies showed the correlation between PE expression and iron metabolism. The *P. aeruginosa* produces pyoverdine to gain iron ions. Some studies claim that iron can lead to the up-regulation of the PE expression by the pyoverdine [101]. On the other hand, *P. aeruginosa* uses glucose to obtain energy. Initially, the glucose oxidizes to 2-ketogluconate in the cytoplasm.

In normal mode, two PtxS that leads to the repression of PE promotor inhibit the transcription of PE. But, 2-ketogluconate can bind to PtxS and dissociate it from PtxR/DNA complex. Therefore, PtxR causes transcription of the toxin by the RNA polymerase [102]. After the production of PE protein, it will be secreted through the T2SS.

The expression of PE protein in the form of unfolded protein is the start point of the intoxication pathway. After that, along the passage of PE precursor through the inner membrane, the signal peptide cleaves and it will enter into the periplasmic space by the Tat system.

Subsequently, the T2SS is located at the outer membrane, so the mature PE protein will cross through the outer membrane by the T2SS. There is a special term XcP in *P. aeruginosa* that is used for the PE protein when it is secreted to the environment. As it is known, many enzymes are present in the host cells that one of them is carboxypeptidase. This enzyme has an important role in the excising of terminal lysine. In the following, the c-terminal motif will form by converting REPLK (aa 609-613) to REDL (aa 609-612). Then, the toxin can bind to KDEL receptor, which is the Golgi/intermediate compartment [103].

Besides, the specific receptor for exotoxin A protein is an alpha2-macroglobulin(α2M). The α2M receptor is a low-density lipoprotein and is mostly produced by the liver. So, the effect of exotin A can be seen on the liver cells frequently. It is encoded by the A2M gene and synthesized by the macrophages, fibroblasts and adrenocortical cells [104]. At the end of this part, the PE protein is faced with two distinct pathways. One of them is KDEL- receptor-mediated pathway and another one is the lipid-dependent sorting pathway, both of them lead to receiving exotoxin A to the Endoplasmatic Reticulum [105].

The α2M is also recognized as CD91 receptor. The exotoxin A binds to the CD91, which is located at the host cell surface and inters to the host cell cytosol *via* Clathrin-Mediated Endocytosis. By the entering of the exotoxin A, the early endosome will be formed that has acidic pH. Then, the PE protein will be disconnected from the CD91 and also a conformational change occurs in its structure. On the other hand, there is a furin motif inside the domain II exotoxin A, which will be cleaved by the protease. The protease enzyme excises the PE protein into two fragments that name R-279 and G-280 [106, 107]. The first fragment belongs to the N-terminus and it has a 28-KDa weight. Another fragment corresponds to the C-terminus of the toxin, which is 37-KDa and consists of domain II and enzymatic domain III. The 37-KDa fragment can be transported to the ER by sec61 complex. There is a special sequence at the c-terminus of the exotoxin A named REDLK (Arg-Glu-Asp-Leu-Lys) that is similar to the KDEL (Lys-Asp-Glu-Leu) motif of the ER [108, 109]. So, the REDLK sequence is a very important component of the intoxication of *P. aeruginosa* [110]. The KDLE may be replaced with C-terminus sequence and obtain much higher toxicity [109].

Eventually, the exotoxin A affects the elongation factor2 (EF2), which leads to inhibition of the protein synthesis [111]. The EF2 translocates the peptidyl-tRNA on the ribosome and causes the production of the peptide chain [112]. Partially, one of the fragments has a crucial role in the activity of the endotoxin A (subunit A) and has ADP- ribosylation activity, which consists of aa 280-613. As was mentioned the exotoxin A reacts with the elongation factor 2 by the ADP-ribosylation reaction. By this process, the EF2 will be inactive that leads to inhibition of protein synthesis in the host cells, and cells go to die. This mechanism also can be seen in diphtheria toxin [113].

5.2. Exotoxin S

In 1978, Barbara H. Iglewski and *et al.* succeeded to differentiate Exotoxin S from Exotoxin A [114].Given the high potential of *P. aeruginosa* virulence, recognition of its pathogenicity factors has high importance.

At the beginning of the infection, *P. aeruginosa* injects several effectors by the type III secretion system into the epithelial cells of the host. These effectors included ExoS, ExoT, ExoU, and ExoY. The ExoS showed more than 50% amino acid homology to Exotoxin A [115]. The cooperation between these two toxins facilitates the replication of the bacteria through changes in the cell structure. Indeed, the N terminus region of the Exotoxin S has GTPase activity and in contrast, the C terminus region has ADP-ribosyltransferase activity. Accordingly, the Exotoxin S is a bifunctional enzyme. So that, the GTPase activity of the Exotoxin S affects the polymerization of the actin and the ADP-ribosyltransferase activity affects Ras- and Rho-family GTPases as well as, ezrin/radixin/moesin proteins [116]. It was suggested that Exotoxin S can be found in strains that are involved in burn infections and contributes to the dissemination of bacteria into the bloodstream [117]. It probably protects the bacteria from being killed by macrophages and PMNs. In addition, it disrupts the host cell membrane [118]. Generally, Exotoxin S has a great role in the pathogenicity of *P. aeruginosa*.

5.3. Leukocidin (Cytotoxin)

A scientist named Scharmann described the leukocidin of *P. aeruginosa* in 1976 [119]. There is a significant similarity between the leukocidin of *P. aeruginosa* with staphylococcal leucocidin [120 - 122]. As the name of this toxin shows, it is effective only on leukocytes but not erythrocytes and thrombocytes [123]. Obviously, it causes morphological alternations in rabbit leukocytes such as leukocytes enlargement and rounded dead cells while the plasma membrane remains intact [123]. The cell-bound protein encodes in the genome of φCTX phage. Then, it will be transferred into the *P. aeruginosa* cells by the phage conversion. Afterward, it will be produced as a protoxin and released during the bacterial lysis [124]. In fact, it is inactive when bounded to the cell. Then, by the lyses of the *P. aeruginosa*, it will be active though the protease digestion. Afterward, it will form hydrophilic pores in the cell membrane of the targeted cells. Lastly, there is a concise site of similarity between mentioned cytotoxic with α-toxin from *Staphylococcus aureus* and aerolysin from *Aeromonas* species [125].

5.4. Enterotoxin

After the injection of the live *P. aeruginosa* into the rabbit, the capacity of this organism to cause fluid accumulation was proven by Kubota *et al.* in 1971. This is a heat-sensitive enterotoxin and could be destroyed by the tyrosine. Although, *P. aeruginosa* is regarded as one of the causes of diarrhea but the amount of the fluid and intensity of its production is much less than *Vibrio Chorea* [126].

6. ENZYMES

6.1. Phospholipase C (PLC)

The PLC is a heat-labile hemolysin and it is involved in *P. aeruginosa* invasion [127]. The PLC causes disruption of phosphorylcholine, which is one of the main components of pulmonary surfactant [126]. Therefore, the surfactant will be lost and atelectasis can happen. In detail, when the alveoli of the lungs filled with the alveolar fluid, the collapse will appear in the whole or some parts of the lungs, which is called atelectasis [128]. In addition, metabolites of the arachidonic acid produced including, prostaglandins, thromboxanes, and leukotrienes [129]. However, osmoprotectors are the most significant products of the PLC and they protect the bacteria from high osmotic pressure of pulmonary environments [130].

The expression of the PLC depends on the mineral phosphate and carbohydrates. So by decreasing the level of the phosphates and carbohydrates, the expression of PLC will be increased [131].

There are two kinds of PLC in *P. aeruginosa*. One of them is named PLC-H and has high molecular weight and it is hemolytic. Another one is PLC-N, which is nonhemolytic with low molecular weight [132]. One of the major aims of PlcH is the degradation of host phospholipids.

This ability may seem to be very helpful in conditions of phosphate starvation but it is not compensatory enough. Interestingly, in addition to phosphate starvation, the PlcHR operon also expresses under the Pi appropriate condition, which can be occurred by the available choline.

On the other hand, as it was mentioned the other extracellular PLC of *P. aeruginosa* is PlcN, which is active on phosphatidylserine but it is not active on sphingomyelin.

There are still some other PLCs in *P. aeruginosa* that PlcB and PlcA can be mentioned among of them [133].

6.2. Rhamnolipid

Rhamnolipid is a kind of bacterial surfactant with amphiphilic properties. As well, there are rhamnose sugars and fatty acids in the structure of this molecule [134]. Rhamnolipid is a kind of bacterial surfactant and *P. aeruginosa* is the most important producer of it. Also, *P. putida* and *P. chlororaphis* and *Burkholderia pseudomallei* can produce rhamnolipids.

However, several functions are defined for the rhamnolipids that we will briefly explain some of them. This molecule forms a hydrophilic surface for the bacterium, which helps *P. aeruginosa* to uptake hydrophobic substrates. In the other form, rhamnolipids can be secreted into the environment by *P. aeruginosa*. Then, the desired substrate can be absorbed much more easily after reacting with rhamnolipids [134, 135].

Another rhamnolipid feature that has been thoroughly proven is its antimicrobial activity against a verity range of microorganisms, from bacteria to fungi including, *Serratia marcescens*, *Klebsiella pneumonia (K. pneumonia)*, *Staphylococcus aureus*, and *Bacillus subtilis, Fusarium solani* and *Penicillium funiculosum* [136].

In addition, rhamnolipid is associated with pulmonary infections, especially in patients with ventilator-associated pneumonia [137]. However, it inhibits the activity of the respiratory ciliates and stimulates mucin secretion in pulmonary infections [138]. On the other hand, rhamnolipid is also involved in the structure of the biofilm. It forms channels that can transfer water and oxygen inside the biofilm structure [139]. This molecule also helps bacteria to fight against the immune system. For this purpose, it kills macrophages and inhibits phagocytosis [140]. Another great property of the rhamnolipid is its ability to maintain infection in cystic fibrosis patients. So that, it causes the demolition of epithelial cells, which leads to increasing of invention, inhibition of mucus cleansing and ciliostasis [138]. Lastly, the rhamnolipid also contributes to swarming motility [141].

6.3. Proteases

6.3.1. LasB

The pathogenic bacteria use various virulence factors to enhance their ability to damage host tissues and develop diseases. LasB is one of the secretable virulence factors of *P. aeruginosa* that can be secreted to the environment by the T2SS [142]. It has an elastic metalloproteinase activity and it is encoded by the *lasB gene* [143]. Therefore, the resulting LasB protein has 33-KDa weight and utilizes calcium ion to be stabilized [144].

Also, it belongs to the thermolysin/M4 peptidase family [122]. The role of LasB has been proven in the biofilm formation and swarming of the *P. aeruginosa* but the main mission of LasB is to facilitate bacterial colonization [145]. Therefore, the expression of lasB increases sharply during the colonization, especially in the lungs. Therefore, it is directly associated with the ventilator-associated pneumonia and causes the pro-inflammatory response. As regards, the pulmonary immune system components are disrupted by the very high toxicity of lasB. In addition, lasB can affect tight junctions, which leads to the destruction of endothelial and epithelial barriers. Finally, lasB causes tissue damage and bacterial elution against the host immune system.

6.3.2. LasA

LasA is a zinc metallopeptidase that is also named as a staphylolysin [146]. It is secreted into the extracellular environment and acts as an elastase and leads to the breakdown of elastin [147, 148]. The elastinolytic property is highly dependent on the function of LasA in *P. aeruginosa* [147]. Accordingly, it mostly affects glycine-glycine bind in the targeted peptide and will hydrolyze it. In addition, LasA is effective on some sites of elastin peptides [149]. On the other hand, lasA has a great role in activating the elastinolytic property of lasB elastase. All of these abilities of LasB lead to break the physical barriers of the host and successful colonization. Furthermore, LasA has other important functions such as tyrosine-kinase activity. In detail, LasA causes shedding of heparin sulfate in the mouse long model, so that, it conquers the cationic antimicrobial peptide, which results to increase of virulence [150].

6.3.3. Alkaline Protease

Alkaline protease, which also called AprA is a zinc metalloprotease and inhibited by chelating factors [151]. It has 50-kDa weight and generally contributes to tissue damage and diffusion. Therefore, AprA affects the development of vascular lesions and necrosis in the cornea [152, 153]. In addition, it disrupts the respiratory system of epithelial cells, which can disorder the cilia movement. Furthermore, another important role of alkaline protease is the suppression of the immune system [36]. Hence, AprA degrades C1q and C3 complement molecules, cytokines, TNF-α and IFN-γ. In parallel, some studies demonstrated that AprA also stops the complement pathway by blocking the classical and lectin pathway [154].

6.3.4. Protease IV

Protease IV is an exoenzyme, which causes particularly disruption of ocular tissue and leads to keratitis. Generally, it can degrade several molecules such as C3, C1q, IgG fibrinogen, plasmin, and plasminogen [155, 156]. The protease IV is approximately 26kDa with 8.7 isoelectric points. In addition, pH 10.0 and 45 °C is appropriate for the best activity of Protease IV [157].

CONSENT FOR PUBLICATION

Not applicable.

CONFLICT OF INTEREST

The authors declare no conflict of interest, financial or otherwise.

ACKNOWLEDGEMENTS

Declared none.

REFERENCES

[1]   Gellatly SL, Hancock RE. *Pseudomonas aeruginosa*: new insights into pathogenesis and host defenses. Pathog Dis 2013; 67(3): 159-73.
       [http://dx.doi.org/10.1111/2049-632X.12033] [PMID: 23620179]

[2]   Byrd MS, Pang B, Mishra M, Swords WE, Wozniak DJ. The *Pseudomonas aeruginosa* exopolysaccharide Psl facilitates surface adherence and NF-kappaB activation in A549 cells. MBio 2010; 1(3): e00140-10.
       [http://dx.doi.org/10.1128/mBio.00140-10] [PMID: 20802825]

[3]   Pier GB. *Pseudomonas aeruginosa* lipopolysaccharide: a major virulence factor, initiator of inflammation and target for effective immunity. Int J Med Microbiol 2007; 297(5): 277-95.
       [http://dx.doi.org/10.1016/j.ijmm.2007.03.012] [PMID: 17466590]

[4]   Li J-D, Dohrman AF, Gallup M, *et al.* Transcriptional activation of mucin by *Pseudomonas aeruginosa* lipopolysaccharide in the pathogenesis of cystic fibrosis lung disease. Proc Natl Acad Sci USA 1997; 94(3): 967-72.
[http://dx.doi.org/10.1073/pnas.94.3.967] [PMID: 9023366]

[5]   Rietschel ET, Kirikae T, Schade FU, *et al.* Bacterial endotoxin: molecular relationships of structure to activity and function. FASEB J 1994; 8(2): 217-25.
[http://dx.doi.org/10.1096/fasebj.8.2.8119492] [PMID: 8119492]

[6]   Schumann RR, Leong SR, Flaggs GW, *et al.* Structure and function of lipopolysaccharide binding protein. Science 1990; 249(4975): 1429-31.
[http://dx.doi.org/10.1126/science.2402637] [PMID: 2402637]

[7]   Erridge C, Bennett-Guerrero E, Poxton IR. Structure and function of lipopolysaccharides. Microbes Infect 2002; 4(8): 837-51.
[http://dx.doi.org/10.1016/S1286-4579(02)01604-0] [PMID: 12270731]

[8]   Alhazmi A. *Pseudomonas aeruginosa*-pathogenesis and pathogenic mechanisms. Int J Biol 2015; 7(2): 44.
[http://dx.doi.org/10.5539/ijb.v7n2p44]

[9]   Shi W, Sun H. Type IV pilus-dependent motility and its possible role in bacterial pathogenesis. Infect Immun 2002; 70(1): 1-4.
[http://dx.doi.org/10.1128/IAI.70.1.1-4.2002] [PMID: 11748156]

[10]   Fletcher M, Savage DC. Bacterial adhesion: mechanisms and physiological significance. Springer Science & Business Media 2013.

[11]   Sharma A, Krause A, Worgall S. Recent developments for Pseudomonas vaccines. Hum Vaccin 2011; 7(10): 999-1011.
[http://dx.doi.org/10.4161/hv.7.10.16369] [PMID: 21941090]

[12]   Hahn HP. The type-4 pilus is the major virulence-associated adhesin of *Pseudomonas aeruginosa*-a review. Gene 1997; 192(1): 99-108.
[http://dx.doi.org/10.1016/S0378-1119(97)00116-9] [PMID: 9224879]

[13]   Klausen M, Heydorn A, Ragas P, *et al.* Biofilm formation by *Pseudomonas aeruginosa* wild type, flagella and type IV pili mutants. Mol Microbiol 2003; 48(6): 1511-24.
[http://dx.doi.org/10.1046/j.1365-2958.2003.03525.x] [PMID: 12791135]

[14]   Leighton TL, Buensuceso RN, Howell PL, Burrows LL. Biogenesis of *Pseudomonas aeruginosa* type IV pili and regulation of their function. Environ Microbiol 2015; 17(11): 4148-63.
[http://dx.doi.org/10.1111/1462-2920.12849] [PMID: 25808785]

[15]   Craig L, Forest KT, Maier B. Type IV pili: dynamics, biophysics and functional consequences. Nat Rev Microbiol 2019; 17(7): 429-40.
[http://dx.doi.org/10.1038/s41579-019-0195-4] [PMID: 30988511]

[16]   Whitchurch CB, Beatson SA, Comolli JC, *et al.* *Pseudomonas aeruginosa* fimL regulates multiple virulence functions by intersecting with Vfr-modulated pathways. Mol Microbiol 2005; 55(5): 1357-78.
[http://dx.doi.org/10.1111/j.1365-2958.2005.04479.x] [PMID: 15720546]

[17]   Semmler AB, Whitchurch CB, Mattick JS. A re-examination of twitching motility in *Pseudomonas aeruginosa*. Microbiology (Reading) 1999; 145(Pt 10): 2863-73.
[http://dx.doi.org/10.1099/00221287-145-10-2863] [PMID: 10537208]

[18]   Wolfgang MC, Lee VT, Gilmore ME, Lory S. Coordinate regulation of bacterial virulence genes by a novel adenylate cyclase-dependent signaling pathway. Dev Cell 2003; 4(2): 253-63.
[http://dx.doi.org/10.1016/S1534-5807(03)00019-4] [PMID: 12586068]

[19] Persat A, Inclan YF, Engel JN, Stone HA, Gitai Z. Type IV pili mechanochemically regulate virulence factors in *Pseudomonas aeruginosa*. Proc Natl Acad Sci USA 2015; 112(24): 7563-8.
[http://dx.doi.org/10.1073/pnas.1502025112] [PMID: 26041805]

[20] Chang C-Y. Surface sensing for biofilm formation in *Pseudomonas aeruginosa*. Front Microbiol 2018; 8: 2671.
[http://dx.doi.org/10.3389/fmicb.2017.02671] [PMID: 29375533]

[21] Rasamiravaka T, Labtani Q, Duez P, El Jaziri M. The formation of biofilms by *Pseudomonas aeruginosa*: a review of the natural and synthetic compounds interfering with control mechanisms. BioMed research international 2015.

[22] McCutcheon JG, Peters DL, Dennis JJ. Identification and characterization of type IV Pili as the cellular receptor of broad host range *Stenotrophomonas maltophilia* bacteriophages DLP1 and DLP2. Viruses 2018; 10(6): 338.
[http://dx.doi.org/10.3390/v10060338] [PMID: 29925793]

[23] de Bentzmann S, Roger P, Dupuit F, *et al.* Asialo GM1 is a receptor for *Pseudomonas aeruginosa* adherence to regenerating respiratory epithelial cells. Infect Immun 1996; 64(5): 1582-8.
[http://dx.doi.org/10.1128/IAI.64.5.1582-1588.1996] [PMID: 8613364]

[24] Avichezer D, Katcoff DJ, Garber NC, Gilboa-Garber N. Analysis of the amino acid sequence of the *Pseudomonas aeruginosa* galactophilic PA-I lectin. J Biol Chem 1992; 267(32): 23023-7.
[http://dx.doi.org/10.1016/S0021-9258(18)50050-8] [PMID: 1429650]

[25] Glick J, Garber N. The intracellular localization of *Pseudomonas aeruginosa* lectins. J Gen Microbiol 1983; 129(10): 3085-90.
[PMID: 6317795]

[26] Grishin AV, Krivozubov MS, Karyagina AS, Gintsburg AL. *Pseudomonas aeruginosa* lectins as targets for novel antibacterials. Acta Naturae 2015; 7(2): 29-41.
[http://dx.doi.org/10.32607/20758251-2015-7-2-29-41] [PMID: 26085942]

[27] Winzer K, Falconer C, Garber NC, Diggle SP, Camara M, Williams P. The *Pseudomonas aeruginosa* lectins PA-IL and PA-IIL are controlled by quorum sensing and by RpoS. J Bacteriol 2000; 182(22): 6401-11.
[http://dx.doi.org/10.1128/JB.182.22.6401-6411.2000] [PMID: 11053384]

[28] Tielker D, Hacker S, Loris R, *et al. Pseudomonas aeruginosa* lectin LecB is located in the outer membrane and is involved in biofilm formation. Microbiology (Reading) 2005; 151(Pt 5): 1313-23.
[http://dx.doi.org/10.1099/mic.0.27701-0] [PMID: 15870442]

[29] Laughlin RS, Musch MW, Hollbrook CJ, Rocha FM, Chang EB, Alverdy JC. The key role of *Pseudomonas aeruginosa* PA-I lectin on experimental gut-derived sepsis. Ann Surg 2000; 232(1): 133-42.
[http://dx.doi.org/10.1097/00000658-200007000-00019] [PMID: 10862206]

[30] Chemani C, Imberty A, de Bentzmann S, *et al.* Role of LecA and LecB lectins in *Pseudomonas aeruginosa*-induced lung injury and effect of carbohydrate ligands. Infect Immun 2009; 77(5): 2065-75.
[http://dx.doi.org/10.1128/IAI.01204-08] [PMID: 19237519]

[31] Sonawane A, Jyot J, Ramphal R. *Pseudomonas aeruginosa* LecB is involved in pilus biogenesis and protease IV activity but not in adhesion to respiratory mucins. Infect Immun 2006; 74(12): 7035-9.
[http://dx.doi.org/10.1128/IAI.00551-06] [PMID: 17015462]

[32] Herzberg M, Rezene TZ, Ziemba C, Gillor O, Mathee K. Impact of higher alginate expression on deposition of *Pseudomonas aeruginosa* in radial stagnation point flow and reverse osmosis systems. Environ Sci Technol 2009; 43(19): 7376-83.
[http://dx.doi.org/10.1021/es901095u] [PMID: 19848149]

[33]   Evans LR, Linker A. Production and characterization of the slime polysaccharide of *Pseudomonas aeruginosa*. J Bacteriol 1973; 116(2): 915-24.
[http://dx.doi.org/10.1128/JB.116.2.915-924.1973] [PMID: 4200860]

[34]   Peteiro C. Alginate production from marine macroalgae, with emphasis on kelp farming. Alginates and Their Biomedical Applications 2018; 27-66.

[35]   Fett WF, Wells JM, Cescutti P, Wijey C. Identification of exopolysaccharides produced by fluorescent pseudomonads associated with commercial mushroom (*Agaricus bisporus*) production. Appl Environ Microbiol 1995; 61(2): 513-7.
[http://dx.doi.org/10.1128/AEM.61.2.513-517.1995] [PMID: 7574589]

[36]   Govan JR, Fyfe JA, Jarman TR. Isolation of alginate-producing mutants of *Pseudomonas fluorescens*, *Pseudomonas putida* and *Pseudomonas mendocina*. J Gen Microbiol 1981; 125(1): 217-20.
[PMID: 6801192]

[37]   Muhammadi AN, Ahmed N. Genetics of bacterial alginate: alginate genes distribution, organization and biosynthesis in bacteria. Curr Genomics 2007; 8(3): 191-202.
[http://dx.doi.org/10.2174/138920207780833810] [PMID: 18645604]

[38]   Pedersen SS, Høiby N, Espersen F, Koch C. Role of alginate in infection with mucoid *Pseudomonas aeruginosa* in cystic fibrosis. Thorax 1992; 47(1): 6-13.
[http://dx.doi.org/10.1136/thx.47.1.6] [PMID: 1539148]

[39]   Cotton LA, Graham RJ, Lee RJ. The role of alginate in *P. aeruginosa* PAO1 biofilm structural resistance to gentamicin and ciprofloxacin. J Exp Microbiol Immunol 2009; 13: 58-62.

[40]   Stapper AP, Narasimhan G, Ohman DE, *et al.* Alginate production affects *Pseudomonas aeruginosa* biofilm development and architecture, but is not essential for biofilm formation. J Med Microbiol 2004; 53(Pt 7): 679-90.
[http://dx.doi.org/10.1099/jmm.0.45539-0] [PMID: 15184541]

[41]   Orgad O, Oren Y, Walker SL, Herzberg M. The role of alginate in *Pseudomonas aeruginosa* EPS adherence, viscoelastic properties and cell attachment. Biofouling 2011; 27(7): 787-98.
[http://dx.doi.org/10.1080/08927014.2011.603145] [PMID: 21797737]

[42]   Lovewell RR, Patankar YR, Berwin B. Mechanisms of phagocytosis and host clearance of *Pseudomonas aeruginosa*. Am J Physiol Lung Cell Mol Physiol 2014; 306(7): L591-603.
[http://dx.doi.org/10.1152/ajplung.00335.2013] [PMID: 24464809]

[43]   Feldman M, Bryan R, Rajan S, *et al.* Role of flagella in pathogenesis of *Pseudomonas aeruginosa* pulmonary infection. Infect Immun 1998; 66(1): 43-51.
[http://dx.doi.org/10.1128/IAI.66.1.43-51.1998] [PMID: 9423837]

[44]   Ramphal R, Sadoff JC, Pyle M, Silipigni JD. Role of pili in the adherence of *Pseudomonas aeruginosa* to injured tracheal epithelium. Infect Immun 1984; 44(1): 38-40.
[http://dx.doi.org/10.1128/IAI.44.1.38-40.1984] [PMID: 6142863]

[45]   Woods DE, Straus DC, Johanson WG Jr, Berry VK, Bass JA. Role of pili in adherence of *Pseudomonas aeruginosa* to mammalian buccal epithelial cells. Infect Immun 1980; 29(3): 1146-51.
[PMID: 6107276]

[46]   Balloy V, Verma A, Kuravi S, Si-Tahar M, Chignard M, Ramphal R. The role of flagellin *versus* motility in acute lung disease caused by *Pseudomonas aeruginosa*. J Infect Dis 2007; 196(2): 289-96.
[http://dx.doi.org/10.1086/518610] [PMID: 17570117]

[47]   Stocker R, Seymour JR. Ecology and physics of bacterial chemotaxis in the ocean. Microbiol Mol Biol Rev 2012; 76(4): 792-812.
[http://dx.doi.org/10.1128/MMBR.00029-12] [PMID: 23204367]

[48]   Verma A, Arora SK, Kuravi SK, Ramphal R. Roles of specific amino acids in the N terminus of *Pseudomonas aeruginosa* flagellin and of flagellin glycosylation in the innate immune response. Infect

Immun 2005; 73(12): 8237-46.
[http://dx.doi.org/10.1128/IAI.73.12.8237-8246.2005] [PMID: 16299320]

[49]   Ringel MT, Brüser T. The biosynthesis of pyoverdines. Microb Cell 2018; 5(10): 424-37.
[http://dx.doi.org/10.15698/mic2018.10.649] [PMID: 30386787]

[50]   Cézard C, Farvacques N, Sonnet P. Chemistry and biology of pyoverdines, Pseudomonas primary
siderophores. Curr Med Chem 2015; 22(2): 165-86.
[http://dx.doi.org/10.2174/0929867321666141011194624] [PMID: 25312210]

[51]   Poole K, Zhao Q, Neshat S, Heinrichs DE, Dean CR. The *Pseudomonas aeruginosa* tonB gene
encodes a novel TonB protein. Microbiology (Reading) 1996; 142(Pt 6): 1449-58.
[http://dx.doi.org/10.1099/13500872-142-6-1449] [PMID: 8704984]

[52]   Skaar EP. The battle for iron between bacterial pathogens and their vertebrate hosts. PLoS Pathog
2010; 6(8): e1000949.
[http://dx.doi.org/10.1371/journal.ppat.1000949] [PMID: 20711357]

[53]   Pierson LS III, Pierson EA. Metabolism and function of phenazines in bacteria: impacts on the
behavior of bacteria in the environment and biotechnological processes. Appl Microbiol Biotechnol
2010; 86(6): 1659-70.
[http://dx.doi.org/10.1007/s00253-010-2509-3] [PMID: 20352425]

[54]   Hall S, McDermott C, Anoopkumar-Dukie S, *et al.* Cellular effects of pyocyanin, a secreted virulence
factor of *Pseudomonas aeruginosa*. Toxins (Basel) 2016; 8(8): 236.
[http://dx.doi.org/10.3390/toxins8080236] [PMID: 27517959]

[55]   Leidal KG, Munson KL, Denning GM. Small molecular weight secretory factors from *Pseudomonas
aeruginosa* have opposite effects on IL-8 and RANTES expression by human airway epithelial cells.
Am J Respir Cell Mol Biol 2001; 25(2): 186-95.
[http://dx.doi.org/10.1165/ajrcmb.25.2.4273] [PMID: 11509328]

[56]   Ran H, Hassett DJ, Lau GW. Human targets of *Pseudomonas aeruginosa* pyocyanin. Proc Natl Acad
Sci USA 2003; 100(24): 14315-20.
[http://dx.doi.org/10.1073/pnas.2332354100] [PMID: 14605211]

[57]   Wilson R, Sykes DA, Watson D, Rutman A, Taylor GW, Cole PJ. Measurement of *Pseudomonas
aeruginosa* phenazine pigments in sputum and assessment of their contribution to sputum sol toxicity
for respiratory epithelium. Infect Immun 1988; 56(9): 2515-7.
[http://dx.doi.org/10.1128/IAI.56.9.2515-2517.1988] [PMID: 3137173]

[58]   McDermott C, Chess-Williams R, Grant GD, *et al.* Effects of *Pseudomonas aeruginosa* virulence
factor pyocyanin on human urothelial cell function and viability. J Urol 2012; 187(3): 1087-93.
[http://dx.doi.org/10.1016/j.juro.2011.10.129] [PMID: 22266010]

[59]   McFarland AJ, Anoopkumar-Dukie S, Perkins AV, Davey AK, Grant GD. Inhibition of autophagy by
3-methyladenine protects 1321N1 astrocytoma cells against pyocyanin- and 1-hydroxyphenazin-
-induced toxicity. Arch Toxicol 2012; 86(2): 275-84.
[http://dx.doi.org/10.1007/s00204-011-0755-5] [PMID: 21964636]

[60]   Poore S, Berry B, Eidson D, McKie KT, Harris RA. Evidence of vascular endothelial dysfunction in
young patients with cystic fibrosis. Chest 2013; 143(4): 939-45.
[http://dx.doi.org/10.1378/chest.12-1934] [PMID: 23099448]

[61]   Cheluvappa R, Jamieson HA, Hilmer SN, Muller M, Le Couteur DG. The effect of *Pseudomonas
aeruginosa* virulence factor, pyocyanin, on the liver sinusoidal endothelial cell. J Gastroenterol
Hepatol 2007; 22(8): 1350-1.
[http://dx.doi.org/10.1111/j.1440-1746.2007.05016.x] [PMID: 17688676]

[62]   Boquist L, Boström T. Alloxan effects on mitochondria *in vitro*, studied with regard to inhibition of
mitochondrial aconitase. Diabete Metab 1985; 11(4): 232-7.
[PMID: 4043490]

[63]   O'Malley YQ, Abdalla MY, McCormick ML, Reszka KJ, Denning GM, Britigan BE. Subcellular localization of Pseudomonas pyocyanin cytotoxicity in human lung epithelial cells. Am J Physiol Lung Cell Mol Physiol 2003; 284(2): L420-30.
        [http://dx.doi.org/10.1152/ajplung.00316.2002] [PMID: 12414438]

[64]   Johnson DI. Beck Bacterial pathogens and their virulence factors. Springer 2018.
        [http://dx.doi.org/10.1007/978-3-319-67651-7]

[65]   Schieber M, Chandel NS. ROS function in redox signaling and oxidative stress. Curr Biol 2014; 24(10): R453-62.
        [http://dx.doi.org/10.1016/j.cub.2014.03.034] [PMID: 24845678]

[66]   Ogunnariwo J, Hamilton-Miller JM. Brown- and red-pigmented *Pseudomonas aeruginosa*: differentiation between melanin and pyorubrin. J Med Microbiol 1975; 8(1): 199-203.
        [http://dx.doi.org/10.1099/00222615-8-1-199] [PMID: 805242]

[67]   Hocquet D, Petitjean M, Rohmer L, *et al.* Pyomelanin-producing *Pseudomonas aeruginosa* selected during chronic infections have a large chromosomal deletion which confers resistance to pyocins. Environ Microbiol 2016; 18(10): 3482-93.
        [http://dx.doi.org/10.1111/1462-2920.13336] [PMID: 27119970]

[68]   Turick CE, Knox AS, Becnel JM, Ekechukwu AA, Milliken CE. Properties and function of pyomelanin. Biopolymers 2010; 449: 72.

[69]   Rodríguez-Rojas A, Mena A, Martín S, Borrell N, Oliver A, Blázquez J. Inactivation of the hmgA gene of *Pseudomonas aeruginosa* leads to pyomelanin hyperproduction, stress resistance and increased persistence in chronic lung infection. Microbiology (Reading) 2009; 155(Pt 4): 1050-7.
        [http://dx.doi.org/10.1099/mic.0.024745-0] [PMID: 19332807]

[70]   Cowan ST. Cowan and Steel's manual for the identification of medical bacteria. Cambridge university press 2004.

[71]   Stanier RY, Palleroni NJ, Doudoroff M. The aerobic pseudomonads a taxonomic study. Microbiology 1966; 43(2): 159-271.

[72]   Furukawa S, Kuchma SL, O'Toole GA. Keeping their options open: acute *versus* persistent infections. J Bacteriol 2006; 188(4): 1211-7.
        [http://dx.doi.org/10.1128/JB.188.4.1211-1217.2006] [PMID: 16452401]

[73]   Hentzer á, Eberl á, Givskov á. Transcriptome analysis of *Pseudomonas aeruginosa* biofilm development: anaerobic respiration and iron limitation. Biofilms 2005; 2(1): 37-61.
        [http://dx.doi.org/10.1017/S1479050505001699]

[74]   Flemming H-C, Neu TR, Wozniak DJ. The EPS matrix: the "house of biofilm cells". J Bacteriol 2007; 189(22): 7945-7.
        [http://dx.doi.org/10.1128/JB.00858-07] [PMID: 17675377]

[75]   Sutherland I. Biofilm exopolysaccharides: a strong and sticky framework. Microbiology (Reading) 2001; 147(Pt 1): 3-9.
        [http://dx.doi.org/10.1099/00221287-147-1-3] [PMID: 11160795]

[76]   Franklin MJ, Nivens DE, Weadge JT, Howell PL. Biosynthesis of the *Pseudomonas aeruginosa* extracellular polysaccharides, alginate, Pel, and Psl. Front Microbiol 2011; 2: 167.
        [http://dx.doi.org/10.3389/fmicb.2011.00167] [PMID: 21991261]

[77]   Mulcahy H, Charron-Mazenod L, Lewenza S. *Pseudomonas aeruginosa* produces an extracellular deoxyribonuclease that is required for utilization of DNA as a nutrient source. Environ Microbiol 2010; 12(6): 1621-9.
        [PMID: 20370819]

[78]   Costerton JW, Stewart PS, Greenberg EP. Bacterial biofilms: a common cause of persistent infections. Science 1999; 284(5418): 1318-22.

[http://dx.doi.org/10.1126/science.284.5418.1318] [PMID: 10334980]

[79]   Nadell CD, Xavier JB, Levin SA, Foster KR. The evolution of quorum sensing in bacterial biofilms. PLoS Biol 2008; 6(1): e14.
[http://dx.doi.org/10.1371/journal.pbio.0060014] [PMID: 18232735]

[80]   Ng W-L, Bassler BL. Bacterial quorum-sensing network architectures. Annu Rev Genet 2009; 43: 197-222.
[http://dx.doi.org/10.1146/annurev-genet-102108-134304] [PMID: 19686078]

[81]   Jimenez PN, Koch G, Thompson JA, Xavier KB, Cool RH, Quax WJ. The multiple signaling systems regulating virulence in *Pseudomonas aeruginosa*. Microbiol Mol Biol Rev 2012; 76(1): 46-65.
[http://dx.doi.org/10.1128/MMBR.05007-11] [PMID: 22390972]

[82]   Parsek MR, Greenberg EP. Sociomicrobiology: the connections between quorum sensing and biofilms. Trends Microbiol 2005; 13(1): 27-33.
[http://dx.doi.org/10.1016/j.tim.2004.11.007] [PMID: 15639629]

[83]   Gilbert KB, Kim TH, Gupta R, Greenberg EP, Schuster M. Global position analysis of the *Pseudomonas aeruginosa* quorum-sensing transcription factor LasR. Mol Microbiol 2009; 73(6): 1072-85.
[http://dx.doi.org/10.1111/j.1365-2958.2009.06832.x] [PMID: 19682264]

[84]   Burrows LL. *Pseudomonas aeruginosa* twitching motility: type IV pili in action. Annu Rev Microbiol 2012; 66: 493-520.
[http://dx.doi.org/10.1146/annurev-micro-092611-150055] [PMID: 22746331]

[85]   Schooling S, Charaf U, Allison D, Gilbert P. A role for rhamnolipid in biofilm dispersion. Biofilms 2004; 1(2): 91-9.
[http://dx.doi.org/10.1017/S147905050400119X]

[86]   Rodrigue A, Quentin Y, Lazdunski A, Méjean V, Foglino M. Two-component systems in *Pseudomonas aeruginosa*: why so many? Trends Microbiol 2000; 8(11): 498-504.
[http://dx.doi.org/10.1016/S0966-842X(00)01833-3] [PMID: 11121759]

[87]   Stewart V. Bacterial two-component regulatory systems. Molecular Microbiology 1998; 141-57.

[88]   Parkins MD, Ceri H, Storey DG. *Pseudomonas aeruginosa* GacA, a factor in multihost virulence, is also essential for biofilm formation. Mol Microbiol 2001; 40(5): 1215-26.
[http://dx.doi.org/10.1046/j.1365-2958.2001.02469.x] [PMID: 11401724]

[89]   Kong W, Chen L, Zhao J, *et al.* Hybrid sensor kinase PA1611 in *Pseudomonas aeruginosa* regulates transitions between acute and chronic infection through direct interaction with RetS. Mol Microbiol 2013; 88(4): 784-97.
[http://dx.doi.org/10.1111/mmi.12223] [PMID: 23560772]

[90]   Ventre I, Goodman AL, Vallet-Gely I, *et al.* Multiple sensors control reciprocal expression of *Pseudomonas aeruginosa* regulatory RNA and virulence genes. Proc Natl Acad Sci USA 2006; 103(1): 171-6.
[http://dx.doi.org/10.1073/pnas.0507407103] [PMID: 16373506]

[91]   Rasamiravaka T, Labtani Q, Duez P, El Jaziri M. The formation of biofilms by *Pseudomonas aeruginosa*: a review of the natural and synthetic compounds interfering with control mechanisms. BioMed Res Int 2015; 2015: 759348.
[http://dx.doi.org/10.1155/2015/759348] [PMID: 25866808]

[92]   Merighi M, Lee VT, Hyodo M, Hayakawa Y, Lory S. The second messenger bis-(3'-5')-cyclic-GMP and its PilZ domain-containing receptor Alg44 are required for alginate biosynthesis in *Pseudomonas aeruginosa*. Mol Microbiol 2007; 65(4): 876-95.
[http://dx.doi.org/10.1111/j.1365-2958.2007.05817.x] [PMID: 17645452]

[93]   Hengge R. Principles of c-di-GMP signalling in bacteria. Nat Rev Microbiol 2009; 7(4): 263-73.
[http://dx.doi.org/10.1038/nrmicro2109] [PMID: 19287449]

[94]   Lee VT, Matewish JM, Kessler JL, Hyodo M, Hayakawa Y, Lory S. A cyclic-di-GMP receptor required for bacterial exopolysaccharide production. Mol Microbiol 2007; 65(6): 1474-84.
[http://dx.doi.org/10.1111/j.1365-2958.2007.05879.x] [PMID: 17824927]

[95]   Liu PV. Extracellular toxins of *Pseudomonas aeruginosa*. J Infect Dis 1974; 130(0) (Suppl.): S94-9.
[http://dx.doi.org/10.1093/infdis/130.Supplement.S94] [PMID: 4370620]

[96]   Wedekind JE, Trame CB, Dorywalska M, *et al.* Refined crystallographic structure of *Pseudomonas aeruginosa* exotoxin A and its implications for the molecular mechanism of toxicity. J Mol Biol 2001; 314(4): 823-37.
[http://dx.doi.org/10.1006/jmbi.2001.5195] [PMID: 11734000]

[97]   Gray GL, Smith DH, Baldridge JS, *et al.* Cloning, nucleotide sequence, and expression in Escherichia coli of the exotoxin A structural gene of *Pseudomonas aeruginosa*. Proc Natl Acad Sci USA 1984; 81(9): 2645-9.
[http://dx.doi.org/10.1073/pnas.81.9.2645] [PMID: 6201861]

[98]   Allured VS, Collier RJ, Carroll SF, McKay DB. Structure of exotoxin A of *Pseudomonas aeruginosa* at 3.0-Angstrom resolution. Proc Natl Acad Sci USA 1986; 83(5): 1320-4.
[http://dx.doi.org/10.1073/pnas.83.5.1320] [PMID: 3006045]

[99]   Siegall CB, Chaudhary VK, FitzGerald DJ, Pastan I. Functional analysis of domains II, Ib, and III of Pseudomonas exotoxin. J Biol Chem 1989; 264(24): 14256-61.
[http://dx.doi.org/10.1016/S0021-9258(18)71671-2] [PMID: 2503515]

[100]   Michalska M, Wolf P. Pseudomonas Exotoxin A: optimized by evolution for effective killing. Front Microbiol 2015; 6: 963.
[http://dx.doi.org/10.3389/fmicb.2015.00963] [PMID: 26441897]

[101]   Hunt TA, Peng W-T, Loubens I, Storey DG. The *Pseudomonas aeruginosa* alternative sigma factor PvdS controls exotoxin A expression and is expressed in lung infections associated with cystic fibrosis. Microbiology (Reading) 2002; 148(Pt 10): 3183-93.
[http://dx.doi.org/10.1099/00221287-148-10-3183] [PMID: 12368452]

[102]   Daddaoua A, Fillet S, Fernández M, Udaondo Z, Krell T, Ramos JL. Genes for carbon metabolism and the ToxA virulence factor in *Pseudomonas aeruginosa* are regulated through molecular interactions of PtxR and PtxS. PLoS One 2012; 7(7): e39390.
[http://dx.doi.org/10.1371/journal.pone.0039390] [PMID: 22844393]

[103]   Hessler JL, Kreitman RJ. An early step in Pseudomonas exotoxin action is removal of the terminal lysine residue, which allows binding to the KDEL receptor. Biochem 1997; 36(47): 14577-82.
[http://dx.doi.org/10.1021/bi971447w] [PMID: 9398176]

[104]   Capitani M, Sallese M. The KDEL receptor: new functions for an old protein. FEBS Lett 2009; 583(23): 3863-71.
[http://dx.doi.org/10.1016/j.febslet.2009.10.053] [PMID: 19854180]

[105]   Kounnas MZ, Morris RE, Thompson MR, FitzGerald DJ, Strickland DK, Saelinger CB. The alpha 2-macroglobulin receptor/low density lipoprotein receptor-related protein binds and internalizes Pseudomonas exotoxin A. J Biol Chem 1992; 267(18): 12420-3.
[http://dx.doi.org/10.1016/S0021-9258(18)42291-0] [PMID: 1618748]

[106]   Alami M, Taupiac M-P, Reggio H, Bienvenüe A, Beaumelle B. Involvement of ATP-dependent Pseudomonas exotoxin translocation from a late recycling compartment in lymphocyte intoxication procedure. Mol Biol Cell 1998; 9(2): 387-402.
[http://dx.doi.org/10.1091/mbc.9.2.387] [PMID: 9450963]

[107]   Méré J, Morlon-Guyot J, Bonhoure A, Chiche L, Beaumelle B. Acid-triggered membrane insertion of Pseudomonas exotoxin A involves an original mechanism based on pH-regulated tryptophan exposure. J Biol Chem 2005; 280(22): 21194-201.
[http://dx.doi.org/10.1074/jbc.M412656200] [PMID: 15799975]

[108] Scheel AA, Pelham HR. Identification of amino acids in the binding pocket of the human KDEL receptor. J Biol Chem 1998; 273(4): 2467-72.
[http://dx.doi.org/10.1074/jbc.273.4.2467] [PMID: 9442098]

[109] Seetharam S, Chaudhary VK, FitzGerald D, Pastan I. Increased cytotoxic activity of Pseudomonas exotoxin and two chimeric toxins ending in KDEL. J Biol Chem 1991; 266(26): 17376-81.
[http://dx.doi.org/10.1016/S0021-9258(19)47383-3] [PMID: 1910044]

[110] Chaudhary VK, Jinno Y, FitzGerald D, Pastan I. Pseudomonas exotoxin contains a specific sequence at the carboxyl terminus that is required for cytotoxicity. Proc Natl Acad Sci USA 1990; 87(1): 308-12.
[http://dx.doi.org/10.1073/pnas.87.1.308] [PMID: 2104981]

[111] McEwan DL, Kirienko NV, Ausubel FM. Host translational inhibition by *Pseudomonas aeruginosa* Exotoxin A Triggers an immune response in Caenorhabditis elegans. Cell Host Microbe 2012; 11(4): 364-74.
[http://dx.doi.org/10.1016/j.chom.2012.02.007] [PMID: 22520464]

[112] Moldave K. Eukaryotic protein synthesis. Annu Rev Biochem 1985; 54(1): 1109-49.
[http://dx.doi.org/10.1146/annurev.bi.54.070185.005333] [PMID: 3896117]

[113] Mateyak MK, Kinzy TG. ADP-ribosylation of translation elongation factor 2 by diphtheria toxin in yeast inhibits translation and cell separation. J Biol Chem 2013; 288(34): 24647-55.
[http://dx.doi.org/10.1074/jbc.M113.488783] [PMID: 23853096]

[114] Iglewski BH, Sadoff J, Bjorn MJ, Maxwell ES. *Pseudomonas aeruginosa* exoenzyme S: an adenosine diphosphate ribosyltransferase distinct from toxin A. Proc Natl Acad Sci USA 1978; 75(7): 3211-5.
[http://dx.doi.org/10.1073/pnas.75.7.3211] [PMID: 210453]

[115] Krueger KM, Barbieri JT. The family of bacterial ADP-ribosylating exotoxins. Clin Microbiol Rev 1995; 8(1): 34-47.
[http://dx.doi.org/10.1128/CMR.8.1.34] [PMID: 7704894]

[116] Hauser AR. The type III secretion system of *Pseudomonas aeruginosa*: infection by injection. Nat Rev Microbiol 2009; 7(9): 654-65.
[http://dx.doi.org/10.1038/nrmicro2199] [PMID: 19680249]

[117] Zhapouni A, Farshad S, Alborzi A. *Pseudomonas aeruginosa*: Burn infection. Treatment and antibacterial resistance. Iranian Red Crescent Medical Journal 2009; 11(3)

[118] Rocha CL, Coburn J, Rucks EA, Olson JC. Characterization of *Pseudomonas aeruginosa* exoenzyme S as a bifunctional enzyme in J774A.1 macrophages. Infect Immun 2003; 71(9): 5296-305.
[http://dx.doi.org/10.1128/IAI.71.9.5296-5305.2003] [PMID: 12933877]

[119] Scharmann W. Formation and isolation of leucocidin from *Pseudomonas aeruginosa*. J Gen Microbiol 1976; 93(2): 283-91.
[http://dx.doi.org/10.1099/00221287-93-2-283] [PMID: 6621]

[120] Noda M, Hirayama T, Kato I, Matsuda F. Crystallization and properties of staphylococcal leukocidin. Biochimica et Biophysica Acta (BBA)-. General Subjects 1980; 633(1): 33-44.
[http://dx.doi.org/10.1016/0304-4165(80)90035-5]

[121] Noda M, Kato I, Hirayama T, Matsuda F. Mode of action of staphylococcal leukocidin: effects of the S and F components on the activities of membrane-associated enzymes of rabbit polymorphonuclear leukocytes. Infect Immun 1982; 35(1): 38-45.
[http://dx.doi.org/10.1128/IAI.35.1.38-45.1982] [PMID: 6274802]

[122] Woodin A. Microbial Toxins. New York: Academic Press 1970; Vol. III.

[123] Scharmann W. Purification and characterization of leucocidin from *Pseudomonas aeruginosa*. J Gen Microbiol 1976; 93(2): 292-302.
[http://dx.doi.org/10.1099/00221287-93-2-292] [PMID: 819616]

[124] Nakayama K, Kanaya S, Ohnishi M, Terawaki Y, Hayashi T. The complete nucleotide sequence of φ CTX, a cytotoxin-converting phage of *Pseudomonas aeruginosa*: implications for phage evolution and horizontal gene transfer *via* bacteriophages. Mol Microbiol 1999; 31(2): 399-419.
[http://dx.doi.org/10.1046/j.1365-2958.1999.01158.x] [PMID: 10027959]

[125] Sliwinski-Korell A, Engelhardt H, Kampka M, Lutz F. Oligomerization and structural changes of the pore-forming *Pseudomonas aeruginosa* cytotoxin. Eur J Biochem 1999; 265(1): 221-30.
[http://dx.doi.org/10.1046/j.1432-1327.1999.00718.x] [PMID: 10491177]

[126] Kubota Y, Liu PV. An enterotoxin of *Pseudomonas aeruginosa*. J Infect Dis 1971; 123(1): 97-8.
[http://dx.doi.org/10.1093/infdis/123.1.97] [PMID: 5543221]

[127] Berka RM, Vasil ML. Phospholipase C (heat-labile hemolysin) of *Pseudomonas aeruginosa*: purification and preliminary characterization. J Bacteriol 1982; 152(1): 239-45.
[PMID: 6811552]

[128] Stern RC, Boat TF, Orenstein DM, Wood RE, Matthews LW, Doershuk CF. Treatment and prognosis of lobar and segmental atelectasis in cystic fibrosis. Am Rev Respir Dis 1978; 118(5): 821-6.
[PMID: 736353]

[129] Fick RB Jr. *Pseudomonas aeruginosa* the Opportunist CRC Press 1992.

[130] Fitzsimmons LF, Hampel KJ, Wargo MJ. Cellular choline and glycine betaine pools impact osmoprotection and phospholipase C production in *Pseudomonas aeruginosa*. J Bacteriol 2012; 194(17): 4718-26.
[http://dx.doi.org/10.1128/JB.00596-12] [PMID: 22753069]

[131] Shortridge VD, Lazdunski A, Vasil ML. Osmoprotectants and phosphate regulate expression of phospholipase C in *Pseudomonas aeruginosa*. Mol Microbiol 1992; 6(7): 863-71.
[http://dx.doi.org/10.1111/j.1365-2958.1992.tb01537.x] [PMID: 1602966]

[132] König B, Vasil ML, König W. Role of haemolytic and non-haemolytic phospholipase C from *Pseudomonas aeruginosa* in interleukin-8 release from human monocytes. J Med Microbiol 1997; 46(6): 471-8.
[http://dx.doi.org/10.1099/00222615-46-6-471] [PMID: 9350199]

[133] Pseudomonas RJ. Virulence and gene regulation. Pseudomonas 2004; 2: 1-553.

[134] Desai JD, Banat IM. Microbial production of surfactants and their commercial potential. Microbiol Mol Biol Rev 1997; 61(1): 47-64.
[http://dx.doi.org/10.1128/.61.1.47-64.1997] [PMID: 9106364]

[135] Zhong H, Zeng GM, Yuan XZ, Fu HY, Huang GH, Ren FY. Adsorption of dirhamnolipid on four microorganisms and the effect on cell surface hydrophobicity. Appl Microbiol Biotechnol 2007; 77(2): 447-55.
[http://dx.doi.org/10.1007/s00253-007-1154-y] [PMID: 17899072]

[136] Haba E, Pinazo A, Jauregui O, Espuny MJ, Infante MR, Manresa A. Physicochemical characterization and antimicrobial properties of rhamnolipids produced by *Pseudomonas aeruginosa* 47T2 NCBIM 40044. Biotechnol Bioeng 2003; 81(3): 316-22.
[http://dx.doi.org/10.1002/bit.10474] [PMID: 12474254]

[137] Köhler T, Guanella R, Carlet J, van Delden C. Quorum sensing-dependent virulence during *Pseudomonas aeruginosa* colonisation and pneumonia in mechanically ventilated patients. Thorax 2010; 65(8): 703-10.
[http://dx.doi.org/10.1136/thx.2009.133082] [PMID: 20685744]

[138] Zulianello L, Canard C, Köhler T, Caille D, Lacroix J-S, Meda P. Rhamnolipids are virulence factors that promote early infiltration of primary human airway epithelia by *Pseudomonas aeruginosa*. Infect Immun 2006; 74(6): 3134-47.
[http://dx.doi.org/10.1128/IAI.01772-05] [PMID: 16714541]

[139] Davey ME, Caiazza NC, O'Toole GA. Rhamnolipid surfactant production affects biofilm architecture in *Pseudomonas aeruginosa* PAO1. J Bacteriol 2003; 185(3): 1027-36.
[http://dx.doi.org/10.1128/JB.185.3.1027-1036.2003] [PMID: 12533479]

[140] McClure CD, Schiller NL. Inhibition of macrophage phagocytosis by *Pseudomonas aeruginosa* rhamnolipids *in vitro* and *in vivo*. Curr Microbiol 1996; 33(2): 109-17.
[http://dx.doi.org/10.1007/s002849900084] [PMID: 8662182]

[141] Glick R, Gilmour C, Tremblay J, *et al.* Increase in rhamnolipid synthesis under iron-limiting conditions influences surface motility and biofilm formation in *Pseudomonas aeruginosa*. J Bacteriol 2010; 192(12): 2973-80.
[http://dx.doi.org/10.1128/JB.01601-09] [PMID: 20154129]

[142] Ra'oof WaM. Distribution of algD, lasB, pilB and nan1 genes among MDR clinical isolates of *Pseudomonas aeruginosa* in respect to site of infection. Tikrit Medical Journal 2011; 17(2)

[143] Leduc D, Beaufort N, de Bentzmann S, *et al.* The *Pseudomonas aeruginosa* LasB metalloproteinase regulates the human urokinase-type plasminogen activator receptor through domain-specific endoproteolysis. Infect Immun 2007; 75(8): 3848-58.
[http://dx.doi.org/10.1128/IAI.00015-07] [PMID: 17517866]

[144] Casilag F, Lorenz A, Krueger J, Klawonn F, Weiss S, Häussler S. The LasB elastase of *Pseudomonas aeruginosa* acts in concert with alkaline protease AprA to prevent flagellin-mediated immune recognition. Infect Immun 2015; 84(1): 162-71.
[http://dx.doi.org/10.1128/IAI.00939-15] [PMID: 26502908]

[145] Zhu J, Cai X, Harris TL, *et al.* Disarming *Pseudomonas aeruginosa* virulence factor LasB by leveraging a *Caenorhabditis elegans* infection model. Chem Biol 2015; 22(4): 483-91.
[http://dx.doi.org/10.1016/j.chembiol.2015.03.012] [PMID: 25892201]

[146] Barequet IS, Habot-Wilner Z, Mann O, *et al.* Evaluation of *Pseudomonas aeruginosa* staphylolysin (LasA protease) in the treatment of methicillin-resistant *Staphylococcus aureus* endophthalmitis in a rat model. Graefes Arch Clin Exp Ophthalmol 2009; 247(7): 913-7.
[http://dx.doi.org/10.1007/s00417-009-1061-2] [PMID: 19280208]

[147] Kessler E, Safrin M, Gustin JK, Ohman DE. Elastase and the LasA protease of *Pseudomonas aeruginosa* are secreted with their propeptides. J Biol Chem 1998; 273(46): 30225-31.
[http://dx.doi.org/10.1074/jbc.273.46.30225] [PMID: 9804780]

[148] Ohman DE, Cryz SJ, Iglewski BH. Isolation and characterization of *Pseudomonas aeruginosa* PAO mutant that produces altered elastase. J Bacteriol 1980; 142(3): 836-42.
[http://dx.doi.org/10.1128/JB.142.3.836-842.1980] [PMID: 6769912]

[149] Vessillier S, Delolme F, Bernillon J, Saulnier J, Wallach J. Hydrolysis of glycine-containing elastin pentapeptides by LasA, a metalloelastase from *Pseudomonas aeruginosa*. Eur J Biochem 2001; 268(4): 1049-57.
[http://dx.doi.org/10.1046/j.1432-1327.2001.01967.x] [PMID: 11179971]

[150] Spencer J, Murphy LM, Conners R, Sessions RB, Gamblin SJ. Crystal structure of the LasA virulence factor from *Pseudomonas aeruginosa*: substrate specificity and mechanism of M23 metallopeptidases. J Mol Biol 2010; 396(4): 908-23.
[http://dx.doi.org/10.1016/j.jmb.2009.12.021] [PMID: 20026068]

[151] Maunsell B, Adams C, O'Gara F. Complex regulation of AprA metalloprotease in *Pseudomonas fluorescens* M114: evidence for the involvement of iron, the ECF sigma factor, PbrA and pseudobactin M114 siderophore. Microbiology (Reading) 2006; 152(Pt 1): 29-42.
[http://dx.doi.org/10.1099/mic.0.28379-0] [PMID: 16385113]

[152] Hobden JA. *Pseudomonas aeruginosa* proteases and corneal virulence. DNA Cell Biol 2002; 21(5-6): 391-6.
[http://dx.doi.org/10.1089/10445490260099674] [PMID: 12167241]

[153] Tang A. *Pseudomonas aeruginosa* small protease (PASP): A corneal virulence factor: The University of Mississippi Medical Center 2012.

[154] Laarman AJ, Bardoel BW, Ruyken M, *et al.* *Pseudomonas aeruginosa* alkaline protease blocks complement activation *via* the classical and lectin pathways. J Immunol 2012; 188(1): 386-93.
[http://dx.doi.org/10.4049/jimmunol.1102162] [PMID: 22131330]

[155] Caballero AR, Moreau JM, Engel LS, Marquart ME, Hill JM, O'Callaghan RJ. *Pseudomonas aeruginosa* protease IV enzyme assays and comparison to other Pseudomonas proteases. Anal Biochem 2001; 290(2): 330-7.
[http://dx.doi.org/10.1006/abio.2001.4999] [PMID: 11237336]

[156] Engel LS, Hill JM, Moreau JM, Green LC, Hobden JA, O'Callaghan RJ. *Pseudomonas aeruginosa* protease IV produces corneal damage and contributes to bacterial virulence. Invest Ophthalmol Vis Sci 1998; 39(3): 662-5.
[PMID: 9501882]

[157] Engel LS, Hill JM, Caballero AR, Green LC, O'Callaghan RJ. Protease IV, a unique extracellular protease and virulence factor from *Pseudomonas aeruginosa*. J Biol Chem 1998; 273(27): 16792-7.
[http://dx.doi.org/10.1074/jbc.273.27.16792] [PMID: 9642237]

CHAPTER 4

Epidemiology

M. Mahmoudi[1], S. Ghafourian[1,*], N. Sadeghifard[1] and B. Badaksh[2]

[1] *Department of Microbiology, Faculty of Medicine, Ilam University of Medical Sciences, Ilam, Iran*

[2] *Department of Gastroenterology, Faculty of Medicine, Ilam University of Medical Sciences, Ilam, Iran*

Abstract: One of the most important features of *P. aeruginosa* is its ability to inhabit anywhere, especially in humid environments, which is very important in its dissemination. So, hygiene in public places such as swimming pools or hot tubs can be effective in reducing the incidence of this bacterium. On the other hand, *P. aeruginosa* is one of the main factors of nosocomial infections. Meanwhile, hospitalized patients in intensive care units are at greater risk. Fortunately, *P. aeruginosa* is sensitive to drought, so it is rarely transmitted through surfaces. In contrast, it can be spread through water-related devices such as respiratory therapy equipment, catheters, dialysis tubes, *etc*. *P. aeruginosa* is responsible for 11-13.8% of nosocomial infections including, urinary tract infection, pneumonia, burn wound infection and a blood infection, surgical site infection, *etc*. It is also important in patients with immunedeficiency like those who suffer from cystic fibrosis, severe leukemia, and AIDS. Since *P. aeruginosa* is ubiquitous and opportunistic bacterium, studying its epidemiology can be very effective and helpful in controlling diseases.

Keywords: Cystic fibrosis, Gastrointestinal surgery infection, Immunocompromised patients, Intensive care unit, Nosocomial infection, Pneumonia, Severe burn infection, Urinary tract infection.

P. aeruginosa is an opportunistic pathogen, which is found everywhere abundantly expect less likely in dry surfaces. Accordingly, moist environments are the best places for these bacteria to grow and survive [1]. Given this issue, showers, water baths, hot tubes, sinks, *etc* should be used more carefully [2]. In addition, *P. aeruginosa* can also be found in soil, fresh fruits and vegetables such as agricultural plants [3]. As well, the skin and stool of humans were the habitats of the *P. aeruginosa* [4]. On the other hand, *P. aeruginosa* showed high significance in the health care units, which makes it one of the major nosocomial pathogens

* **Corresponding author S. Ghafourian:** Department of Microbiology, Faculty of Medicine, Ilam University of Medical Sciences, Iran; E-mail: sobhan.ghafurian@gmail.com

worldwide [5] . Therefore , special attention should be paid to respiratory therapy equipment, catheters, dialysis tubing and respiratory devices [6]. Whereas it is sensitive to drought, it cannot be transported through objects in the hospital. But it can be transported through the water that is used to wash medical devices and water of the ornamental as well as equipment that work with water [7, 8].

The high importance of nosocomial infections is due to their high mortality rates [9] so that, approximately 75% of severe nosocomial infections occur in developing countries [10]. However, bacterial pathogens, which can cause nosocomial infections include, *Streptococcus* spp., *Acinetobacter* spp., *enterococci, P. aeruginosa*, coagulase-negative *staphylococci, S. aureus, Bacillus cereus, Legionella, Proteusmirablis, Klebsiella pneumonia, E. coli, Serratia marcescens.* Among the mentioned pathogens, *enterococci, P. aeruginosa, S. aureus,* and *E. coli* are the most prominent [11].

Generally, *P. aeruginosa* accounts for 11-13.8% of nosocomial infections [12, 13]. Hence, urinary tract infection (UTI) is one of the popular hospital-acquired infections that can occur by *P. aeruginosa.* Approximately, *P. aeruginosa* causes 9% of all nosocomial UTIs and specifically, 16.3% UTIs of patients from intensive care units (ICU) [13 - 16]. In addition, using catheters also can cause UTIs. In this case, 10.5% of patients suffer from UTIs while the rate of UTIs in patients who did not use a catheter was 4.1% [17].

Subsequently, whereas *P. aeruginosa* is an opportunistic pathogen, it is extremely problematic in the intensive care units (ICU). Some studies reported that infection with these bacteria is approximately 13.2-22.6% of cases [13, 18, 19].

Despite, *P. aeruginosa* is the second common cause of pneumonia but it is the dominant cause of pediatric ICUs pneumonia [20, 21]. The next significant infection caused by *P. aeruginosa* occurs in patients whom suffer from severe burns and they are already hospitalized [14, 19, 22]. In this case, *P. aeruginosa* is the first cause of lethal infections. Unfortunately, sometimes, the infection spreads *via* bloodstream in patients who are admitted in burn ICUs, which could be extremely dangerous [23].

Lastly, another nosocomial infection caused by *P. aeruginosa* is surgical site infection that allocated 6% of all cases. But in pediatrics ICUs, the range of infection comes almost up, which is approximately 16% [14, 24, 25]. Although the cause of the infection varies among types of surgery, there is a study that presented *P. aeruginosa* as the first cause of infection after gastrointestinal surgery [21].

Also, *P. aeruginosa* has substantial importance in immunosuppression patients such as who has been immunocompromised by congenital or acquired [26]. The reason is the ability of *P. aeruginosa* to act as an opportunistic pathogen and it makes immunosuppression patients a very suitable host [27]. Based on this, in patients suffering from severe leukemia, it can be the cause of bacteremia [28]. As well, AIDS is one of the most well-known immunodeficiency disorders and some of these patients will suffer from pneumonia. The study claimed that *P. aeruginosa* was the most popular bacterium isolated from them [29]. The other cohort study demonstrated that the high-risk patients are those with immunocompromised problems and organ recipients. Therefore, the significantly increased level of the *P. aeruginosa* infection was reported in patients who received organs such as bone marrow/ stem cells, heart, and lung [30, 31]. Diabetic patients also suffer from epidermal necrosis in the food area. Here also, *P. aeruginosa* and *Staphylococcus aureus* isolates from wounds area common cause of infection competitively [32, 33]. Eventually, another group that is at risk of infection with *P. aeruginosa* is cystic fibrosis patients. Based on report of the US Cystic Fibrosis Foundation Patient Registry in 2017, fortunately, the positive culture of *P. aeruginosa* was declined in patients younger than 18 years, so that, the variation range is 47% in 1997 to 27.5% in 2017, but unfortunately, MDR *P. aeruginosa* is still recalcitrant and it is allocated 17.9% positive culture among CF patients during 2017.

Due to the severe pathogenicity of *P. aeruginosa* that can cause and the increasing rate of MDR *P. aeruginosa*, it is suggested that sufficient surveillance should be done on a mentioned group of patients because being aware of its epidemiology can prevent its outbreak properly.

CONSENT FOR PUBLICATION

Not applicable.

CONFLICT OF INTEREST

The authors declare no conflict of interest, financial or otherwise.

ACKNOWLEDGEMENTS

Declared none.

REFERENCES

[1]   Meitert E, Meitert T, Baron E, Sulea I. Distribution in nature of types of *Pseudomonas aeruginosa*. I. Lysotyping of strains of *Pseudomonas aeruginosa* from humans and animals. Arch Roum Pathol Exp Microbiol 1969; 28(4): 957-64.
      [PMID: 4992009]

[2]   Bédard E, Prévost M, Déziel E. *Pseudomonas aeruginosa* in premise plumbing of large buildings. MicrobiologyOpen 2016; 5(6): 937-56.
[http://dx.doi.org/10.1002/mbo3.391] [PMID: 27353357]

[3]   Green SK, Schroth MN, Cho JJ, Kominos SK, Vitanza-jack VB. Agricultural plants and soil as a reservoir for *Pseudomonas aeruginosa*. Appl Microbiol 1974; 28(6): 987-91.
[http://dx.doi.org/10.1128/AM.28.6.987-991.1974] [PMID: 4217591]

[4]   Agger WA, Mardan A. *Pseudomonas aeruginosa* infections of intact skin. Clin Infect Dis 1995; 20(2): 302-8.
[http://dx.doi.org/10.1093/clinids/20.2.302] [PMID: 7742434]

[5]   Khan HA, Ahmad A, Mehboob R. Nosocomial infections and their control strategies. Asian Pac J Trop Biomed 2015; 5(7): 509-14.
[http://dx.doi.org/10.1016/j.apjtb.2015.05.001]

[6]   Carroll KC, Butel J, Morse S. Jawetz Melnick and Adelbergs Medical Microbiology 27 E: McGraw-Hill Education 2015.

[7]   Quick J, Cumley N, Wearn CM, *et al.* Seeking the source of *Pseudomonas aeruginosa* infections in a recently opened hospital: an observational study using whole-genome sequencing. BMJ Open 2014; 4(11): e006278.
[http://dx.doi.org/10.1136/bmjopen-2014-006278] [PMID: 25371418]

[8]   Kerr KG, Snelling AM. *Pseudomonas aeruginosa*: a formidable and ever-present adversary. J Hosp Infect 2009; 73(4): 338-44.
[http://dx.doi.org/10.1016/j.jhin.2009.04.020] [PMID: 19699552]

[9]   Brusaferro S, Arnoldo L, Cattani G, *et al.* Harmonizing and supporting infection control training in Europe. J Hosp Infect 2015; 89(4): 351-6.
[http://dx.doi.org/10.1016/j.jhin.2014.12.005] [PMID: 25777079]

[10]   Obiero CW, Seale AC, Berkley JA. Empiric treatment of neonatal sepsis in developing countries. Pediatr Infect Dis J 2015; 34(6): 659-61.
[http://dx.doi.org/10.1097/INF.0000000000000692] [PMID: 25806843]

[11]   Horan TC, Andrus M, Dudeck MA. CDC/NHSN surveillance definition of health care-associated infection and criteria for specific types of infections in the acute care setting. Am J Infect Control 2008; 36(5): 309-32.
[http://dx.doi.org/10.1016/j.ajic.2008.03.002] [PMID: 18538699]

[12]   Pittet D, Harbarth S, Ruef C, *et al.* Prevalence and risk factors for nosocomial infections in four university hospitals in Switzerland. Infect Control Hosp Epidemiol 1999; 20(1): 37-42.
[http://dx.doi.org/10.1086/501554] [PMID: 9927264]

[13]   Lizioli A, Privitera G, Alliata E, *et al.* Prevalence of nosocomial infections in Italy: result from the Lombardy survey in 2000. J Hosp Infect 2003; 54(2): 141-8.
[http://dx.doi.org/10.1016/S0195-6701(03)00078-1] [PMID: 12818589]

[14]   Gaynes R, Edwards JR, Edwards JR, System NNIS. National Nosocomial Infections Surveillance System. Overview of nosocomial infections caused by gram-negative bacilli. Clin Infect Dis 2005; 41(6): 848-54.
[http://dx.doi.org/10.1086/432803] [PMID: 16107985]

[15]   Chan RK, Lye WC, Lee EJ, Kumarasinghe G. Nosocomial urinary tract infection: a microbiological study. Ann Acad Med Singapore 1993; 22(6): 873-7.
[PMID: 8129347]

[16]   Jodrá VM, Díaz-Agero Pérez C, Sainz de Los Terreros Soler L, Saa Requejo CM, Dacosta Ballesteros D, Group QCIW. Quality Control Indicator Working Group. Results of the Spanish national nosocomial infection surveillance network (VICONOS) for surgery patients from January 1997 through December 2003. Am J Infect Control 2006; 34(3): 134-41.

[http://dx.doi.org/10.1016/j.ajic.2005.10.004] [PMID: 16630977]

[17]   Bouza E, San Juan R, Muñoz P, Voss A, Kluytmans J. Co-operative Group of the European Study Group on Nosocomial Infections; European Study Group on Nosocomial Infections. A European perspective on nosocomial urinary tract infections I. Report on the microbiology workload, etiology and antimicrobial susceptibility (ESGNI-003 study). Clin Microbiol Infect 2001; 7(10): 523-31.
[http://dx.doi.org/10.1046/j.1198-743x.2001.00326.x] [PMID: 11683792]

[18]   Vessillier S, Delolme F, Bernillon J, Saulnier J, Wallach J. Hydrolysis of glycine-containing elastin pentapeptides by LasA, a metalloelastase from *Pseudomonas aeruginosa*. Eur J Biochem 2001; 268(4): 1049-57.
[http://dx.doi.org/10.1046/j.1432-1327.2001.01967.x] [PMID: 11179971]

[19]   Erbay H, Yalcin AN, Serin S, *et al.* Nosocomial infections in intensive care unit in a Turkish university hospital: a 2-year survey. Intensive Care Med 2003; 29(9): 1482-8.
[http://dx.doi.org/10.1007/s00134-003-1788-x] [PMID: 12898002]

[20]   Kollef MH, Shorr A, Tabak YP, Gupta V, Liu LZ, Johannes RS. Epidemiology and outcomes of health-care-associated pneumonia: results from a large US database of culture-positive pneumonia. Chest 2005; 128(6): 3854-62.
[http://dx.doi.org/10.1378/chest.128.6.3854] [PMID: 16354854]

[21]   Richards MJ, Edwards JR, Culver DH, Gaynes RP, System NNIS. Nosocomial infections in pediatric intensive care units in the United States. Pediatrics 1999; 103(4): e39-e.
[http://dx.doi.org/10.1542/peds.103.4.e39]

[22]   Lari AR, Alaghehbandan R. Nosocomial infections in an Iranian burn care center. Burns 2000; 26(8): 737-40.
[http://dx.doi.org/10.1016/S0305-4179(00)00048-6] [PMID: 11024608]

[23]   Taneja N, Emmanuel R, Chari PS, Sharma M. A prospective study of hospital-acquired infections in burn patients at a tertiary care referral centre in North India. Burns 2004; 30(7): 665-9.
[http://dx.doi.org/10.1016/j.burns.2004.02.011] [PMID: 15475139]

[24]   Weiss CA III, Statz CL, Dahms RA, Remucal MJ, Dunn DL, Beilman GJ. Six years of surgical wound infection surveillance at a tertiary care center: review of the microbiologic and epidemiological aspects of 20,007 wounds. Arch Surg 1999; 134(10): 1041-8.
[http://dx.doi.org/10.1001/archsurg.134.10.1041] [PMID: 10522843]

[25]   Arias CA, Quintero G, Vanegas BE, Rico CL, Patiño JF. Surveillance of surgical site infections: decade of experience at a Colombian tertiary care center. World J Surg 2003; 27(5): 529-33.
[http://dx.doi.org/10.1007/s00268-003-6786-1] [PMID: 12715217]

[26]   Chatzinikolaou I, Abi-Said D, Bodey GP, Rolston KV, Tarrand JJ, Samonis G. Recent experience with *Pseudomonas aeruginosa* bacteremia in patients with cancer: Retrospective analysis of 245 episodes. Arch Intern Med 2000; 160(4): 501-9.
[http://dx.doi.org/10.1001/archinte.160.4.501] [PMID: 10695690]

[27]   Bubonja-Sonje M, Matovina M, Skrobonja I, Bedenic B, Abram M. Mechanisms of carbapenem resistance in multidrug-resistant clinical isolates of *Pseudomonas aeruginosa* from a Croatian hospital. Microb Drug Resist 2015; 21(3): 261-9.
[http://dx.doi.org/10.1089/mdr.2014.0172] [PMID: 25565041]

[28]   Funada H, Matsuda T. Changes in the incidence and etiological patterns of bacteremia associated with acute leukemia over a 25-year period. Intern Med 1998; 37(12): 1014-8.
[http://dx.doi.org/10.2169/internalmedicine.37.1014] [PMID: 9932631]

[29]   Vidal F, Mensa J, Martínez JA, *et al. Pseudomonas aeruginosa* bacteremia in patients infected with human immunodeficiency virus type 1. Eur J Clin Microbiol Infect Dis 1999; 18(7): 473-7.
[http://dx.doi.org/10.1007/s100960050326] [PMID: 10482023]

[30]   Lossos IS, Breuer R, Or R, *et al.* Bacterial pneumonia in recipients of bone marrow transplantation. A five-year prospective study. Transplantation 1995; 60(7): 672-8.
[http://dx.doi.org/10.1097/00007890-199510150-00010] [PMID: 7570975]

[31]   Kramer MR, Marshall SE, Starnes VA, Gamberg P, Amitai Z, Theodore J. Infectious complications in heart-lung transplantation. Analysis of 200 episodes. Arch Intern Med 1993; 153(17): 2010-6.
[http://dx.doi.org/10.1001/archinte.1993.00410170090009] [PMID: 8357286]

[32]   Shankar EM, Mohan V, Premalatha G, Srinivasan RS, Usha AR. Bacterial etiology of diabetic foot infections in South India. Eur J Intern Med 2005; 16(8): 567-70.
[http://dx.doi.org/10.1016/j.ejim.2005.06.016] [PMID: 16314237]

[33]   Abdulrazak A, Bitar ZI, Al-Shamali AA, Mobasher LA. Bacteriological study of diabetic foot infections. J Diabetes Complicat 2005; 19(3): 138-41.
[http://dx.doi.org/10.1016/j.jdiacomp.2004.06.001] [PMID: 15866058]

CHAPTER 5

Pathogenicity

M. Mahmoudi[1], S. Ghafourian[1,*], B. Badakhsh[2], H. Kazemian[1] and A. Maleki[3]

[1] *Department of Microbiology, Faculty of Medicine, Ilam University of Medical Sciences, Ilam, Iran*

[2] *Department of Gastroenterology, Faculty of Medicine, Ilam University of Medical Sciences, Ilam, Iran*

[3] *Clinical Microbiology Research Center, Ilam University of Medical Sciences, Ilam, Iran*

Abstract: The importance of understanding the pathogenesis of infectious agents is in the diagnosis of the diseases and finding new treatments. In the case of *P. aeruginosa* pathogenesis, the issue is extremely broad and complex. Also, many aspects of its pathogenesis remain unknown to researchers. At a glance, *P. aeruginosa* causes acute and chronic infections. In addition, *P. aeruginosa* is an opportunistic bacterium that is highly dangerous in immunocompromised patients. In some cases, it can also threaten human life and causes the death of the patients. The ability of *P. aeruginosa* to cross the body barriers is so fascinating, which can penetrate the skin and even depths of the bone and joints. Although the pathogenesis of *P. aeruginosa* depends on many factors, it is attributed to several diseases including, bacteremia, keratitis, pneumonia, bone and joints infection, respiratory tract infection, urinary tract infection, skin and soft tissue infection, ear infection, endocarditis, central nervous system infection, enteric infection, mastitis and, *etc.* The wide range of diseases caused by *P. aeruginosa* clearly demonstrated the importance of this bacterium in the fields of medicine.

Keywords: Acute and chronic infection, Cystic fibrosis, Endocarditis, Opportunistic pathogen, Pathogenicity, Pneumonia, Urinary tract infection.

P. aeruginosa is the cause of various disorders, from acute to chronic infections [1].Given that it is an opportunistic pathogen; it has high importance among patients with immunodeficiency. Furthermore, individuals who suffer from AIDS, organ transplantation, cystic fibrosis and,especially hospitalized patients are at a high risk of various infections by *P. aeruginosa* [2]. In the following, we will explain types of diseases caused by infection with *P. aeruginosa* Fig. (**1**) .

* **Corresponding author S. Ghafourian:** Department of Microbiology, Faculty of Medicine, Ilam University of Medical Sciences, Iran; E-mail: sobhan.ghafurian@gmail.com

Mina Mahmoudi, Sobhan Ghafourian & Behzad Badakhsh (Eds.)
All rights reserved-© 2021 Bentham Science Publishers

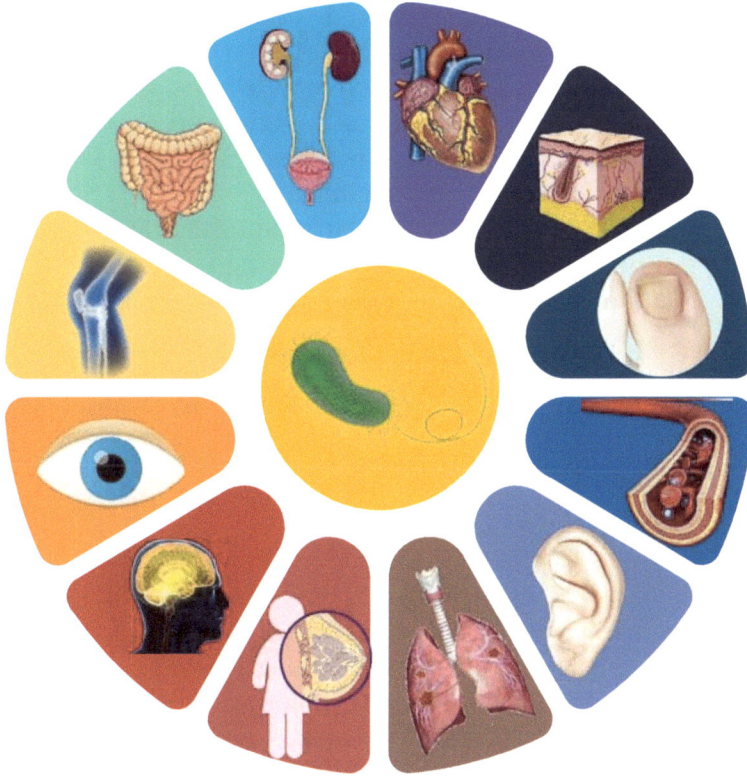

Fig. (1). *P. aeruginosa* pathogenesis. *P. aeruginosa* is responsible for a variety of acute and chronic infections in humans. Infection sites are also very diverse for this bacterium. In short, *P. aeruginosa* can cause bacteremia, keratitis, pneumonia, bone and joints infection, respiratory tract infection, urinary tract infection, skin and soft tissue infection, ear infection, endocarditis, central nervous system infection, enteric infection, mastitis, *etc.*

1. BACTEREMIA

Bacteremia occurs when *P. aeruginosa* succeeds in propagation from the main site of the infection to the bloodstream. For this purpose, it should cross from the tissue barrier of epithelial cells and endothelial cells [3]. In this case, phagocytosis is a very important factor to prevent the dissemination of bacteria into the bloodstream. In addition, complement also plays a role to struggle with the infection but in contrast, *P. aeruginosa* also expresses smooth polysaccharide [4, 5]. In patients with neutropenia, ecthyma gangrenous can occur.

This disorder damages cutaneous tissue and mostly happens in patients who suffer from severe immunodeficiency. The scar caused by ecthyma gangrenous seems to be hemorrhagic and red. Also, the necrotic areas seem to be black [6]. The ecthyma gangrenous can also happen in healthy children less than 1 year but very rarely [7]. In some cases of ecthyma gangrenosum, sepsis also occurs which is very deadly [8]. For instance, according to the studies from 1975 to 2014, among 167 cases, 73.65% (n=123) were positive in terms of *P. aeruginosa*. Besides, 17.35% (n=29) were positive *via* other bacteria including, *E. coli*, *S. aureus*, *Aeromonas hydrophilia,* and *Mucor* species. Out of the 123 patients who had the ecthyma gangrenosum, 58.5% (n=72) suffered from sepsis. There are several factors to cause sepsis leading to death in children. One of the main reasons for associated sepsis mortality by the ecthyma gangrenosum is leukopenia. For instance, it was reported that neutropenia below 500cells/mm3 is strongly associated with *P. aeruginosa* infection that can lead to sepsis and finally death of the patient. The other reason is the postponement of antibiotic therapy [9].This disorder usually occurs due to the activity of protease and elastase of *P. aeruginosa* [10].

2. BONE AND JOINT INFECTIONS

This type of infection is observed very rarely. Usually, *P. aeruginosa* spreads to the bloodstream and then infect the bone and joints or it is arising from adjacent site of infection. Addicts can be infected with unclear intravenous injections or by using contaminated illicit drugs. As well, infective endocarditis are also one of the causes of the distribution of infection into the population of addicts. Unfortunately, these populations probably will suffer from osteomyelitis, septic arthritis and sternoclavicular joint [11]. It is not usually accompanied by fever or it happens with a low grade. People with morphine addiction are more at risk because morphine prevents phagocytosis and inhibits the migration of the neutrophils. In addition to addiction, there are several other risk factors for bone infection by *P. aeruginosa* such as compound fractures, surgery and penetration into wounds deeply [12]. In children *P. aeruginosa* gets access to their wound foot, pain can be felt. Also, another group of patients whose lower limbs are at risk of infection with *P. aeruginosa* is diabetic patients. This infection occurs in patients with chronic or previously treated wounds frequently [13]. There is another bone-associated infection in diabetic or immunocompromised patients named malignant otitis. This infection is also caused by *P. aeruginosa* and destroys the external auditory canal and base of the skull. Although malignant otitis happens very rarely, which is in the category of deadly diseases [14].

3. KERATITIS

Keratitis by *P. aeruginosa* is categorized in the group of medical emergency infections [15]. The reason is the ability to develop and destroyed eyesight. However, one of the most important causes of this infection is using contact lenses that can scratch the cornea. In general, any type of eye trauma can predispose the individual to this infection including, wound or even burn [16, 17]. Some unpopular eye infections occur the following bacteremia *via P. aeruginosa*, for instance, orbital cellulitis and gangrene necrosis of the eyelids [18], but the most horrible effect of this infection is panophthalmit that leads to the loss of sight [19].

4. PNEUMONIA

P. aeruginosa is the first or second cause of ventilator-associated pneumonia with the high mortality range [20]. *P. aeruginosa* is one of the most important pathogens in nosocomial pulmonary infections [21]. One of the most susceptible groups to this kind of pneumonia is cystic fibrosis patients. It is progressive and associated with lung damage [22]. *P. aeruginosa* is not the primary pathogen in cystic fibrosis patients while primary pneumonia is the most commonly seen in patients with cancer and neutropenia [23, 24]. In the mode of secondary infection, initially, the lung is destroyed by other factors such as *S. aureus* or *Haemophilus influenza* [25, 26]. Then, increased proteases in mucin lead to the removal of fibronectin from the surface of epithelial cells. It leads to Ganglioside receptor availability and *P. aeruginosa* can attach to them. In addition, *P. aeruginosa* uses Cystic fibrosis transmembrane conductance regulator as a receptor on epithelial cells and enters into the cells. Besides this, the *P. aeruginosa* can attach to the GM1 *via* pili and flagella [27, 28].

5. CHRONIC RESPIRATORY TRACT INFECTIONS

Chronic infections are usually seen in susceptible individuals or in patients that are not properly treated in the acute phase of the disease. The cystic fibrosis patients are very predisposed to these kinds of respiratory tract infections [11]. In this case, the *P. aeruginosa* will be adapted to the respiratory environment and form the biofilm which leads to the starting of chronic infection. But the cause of this disorder is due to the defects and mutations in some specific receptors including, cystic fibrosis transmembrane regulator (CFTR) [29]. The CFTR acts as a cAMP-dependent chloride channel and mutation causes perturbation of chloride ion secretion. Finally, as the respiratory tract becomes thicker, the mucus becomes unclear and this leads to the remaining of the infection [30]. Accordingly, inflammatory responses occur without interruption that leads to the chronic respiratory tract inflammation [11].

Another chronic infection caused by *P. aeruginosa* is panbronchiolitis and it is mostly reported in Japan [31].The panbronchiolitis is the progressive blocker airway disorder, which is untreatable and may develop to bronchiectasis. Eventually, the respiratory tract will fail and the cause death [32].

6. URINARY TRACT INFECTION (UTI)

20-40% of all nosocomial infections are allocated to UTI and *P. aeruginosa* causes 7-10% of UTI [33], but it can be seen even in non-hospitalized patients, too. In fact, UTI is very common and probably all humans are infected at least once in their lifetime [34, 35]. This infection is more common in women [36]. As well, there are several predisposing factors such as catheters vesicoureteral reflux, surgery, obstruction (for example by kidney stones) diabetes mellitus and organ transplantation [37, 38]. However, the most important of them is using the catheters, which leads to disruption of the mucosal layer of urinary tract. In addition, other pathogens are able to occur catheter-associated UTI such as *E.coli*, *Proteus mirabilis*, *K. pneumoniae* and *Streptococcus faecalis* [39].

7. SKIN AND SOFT TISSUES INFECTIONS

As was mentioned, one of the habitats of *P. aeruginosa* is moisture environments such as skin. Accordingly, there are several different infections in this category. For instance, chronic skin ulcers, burn infections, folliculitis, vesicular lesions, *etc* [20].

In general, approximately 51% of all nosocomial burn infections lead to the death of patients that *S.aureus* is the chair factor of them. Then *Pseudomonas* and *Acinetobacter* are located at the lower scores [40]. Probably, the reason could be uninterrupted increase of antibiotic resistance in *P. aeruginosa*, as well, the misuse and abuse of previous use of antibiotics, the vastness of burn areas and long-term hospitalization are the examples that cause deterioration of infections [41]. By spreading the infection into the bloodstream, fatal bacteremia will occur [42].

The folliculitis is usually obtained from the community and occurs when the hair follicles are contaminated by skin pathogens such as *P. aeruginosa*. It has been proven that hot tubes are highly associated with folliculitis. In addition, there are some other places including, maelstrom, swimming pools, water slides, bathtubs and, *etc* [43].

It may also cause a soldier or athlete's foot infection. This disorder occurs by occlusive footwear such as boots, bandage, or poor quality sneakers. The cleft between thumbs and fourth toes is the most susceptible site for this infection [44].

Among the bacterial pathogens, *P. aeruginosa* is the most common cause of nail infection [45]. It can be recognized by the green color of the nails that happen due to the production of the pyocyanin pigment. Regularly, the infection occurs just in one or two fingers but it is transferable. Other bacteria that can cause nail infection are *Klebsiella* spp. and *S. aureus*. Anyway, the most regular cause of nail infection is dermathophyte [46].

8. EAR INFECTIONS

Swimmer children are one of the susceptible groups due to the lack of complete development of their immune system. This infection usually occurs *via* soaking of the eternal ear canal. Any source of contaminated water, from the artificial pool to the river, can cause infection [20]. Also, this range age has a smaller Eustachian tube compare with older individuals. In some cases, the ear starts draining, which can be yellow or even bloody due to the eardrum rupture [47].

Chronic suppurative otitis media (CSOM) is the most predominant ear infection caused by *P. aeruginosa* in both children and adults. Respiratory tract infection and inappropriate living conditions can predispose the CSOM disorder. Except, *P. aeruginosa*, *S.aureus* is also highly isolated from the culture of CSOM patients [48]. Even though most of the cultures are mixed, but *P. aeruginosa* was the single isolated species in 30% of the cultures [20]. In order to cure this infection, antibiotics should be prescribed with caution. For instance, aminoglycosides are toxic to the inner ear *via* generating free radicals that can cause sensorineural hearingloss, dizziness or tinnitus [49].

9. ENDOCARDITIS

Only 3% of infective endocarditis (IE)is related to the *P. aeruginosa* but it has a high rate of mortality. Almost all the patients used intravenous drugs and approximately just 10% of them did not use [50]. Also, among *P. aeruginosa* IE cases, 70% of them are right-sided [51].

In addicted individuals, the source of the infection usually is the water or material used for the preparation of the drugs. Based on this, the utilization of paraphernalia or illicit drugs is strictly forbidden [11].

Other bacterial causes of IE are *S. aureus*, *Streptococci*, *enterococci*, *Staphylococcus epidermidis*, and the HACEK organisms. Sometimes, the IE occurs in the polymicrobial form that the most popular combination consists of *S.aureus*, *Streptococcus pneumonia* and *P. aeruginosa* [52].

These organisms produce a biofilm that protects them from the immune system of the host and with this manner; it can be easily developed [53].

It should be noted that intravenous drugs are not the only way of contamination but also there are some other ways such as transmission during the surgery process [54].

However, one of the rare complications of this disease is pulmonary embolism, so, only 1.5-2% of all IE cases account for pulmonic endocarditis [55]. In addition, only 3% of *P. aeruginosa* IE cases lead to pulmonary embolism [54].

10. CENTRAL NERVOUS SYSTEM (CNS) INFECTIONS

CNS infection by *P. aeruginosa* usually appears as a secondary infection. So, any lesion or trauma in the head area, surgery or bacteremia can be caused by *P. aeruginosa* CNS infection [20]. *P. aeruginosa* is the most popular nosocomial spontaneous Gram-negative bacillary that causes meningitis and can lead to trismus (dysfunction of the trigeminal nerve, which reduces jaw opening) [56, 57]. In some intravenous drug-addicted cases, secondary brain abscess is also reported [58]. In addition, epidural and subdural empyema also can be associated with *P. aeruginosa* infection [59, 60].

11. ENTERIC INFECTION

Shanghai fever is an enteric infection that is associated with fever, diarrhea and, sepsis [61].

In addition, rose-colored spotted rash also can be seen that is similar to typhoid [62]. It is highly deadly due to the abrupt septic shock and disruption of organs. Also, it is commonly seen in tropical regions such as Taiwan, Hong Kong and China [63].

12. MASTITIS

The disease is usually seen in cattle that causes inflammation in mammary glands [64]. Sometimes, the disease can get worse with the appearance of necrosis and gangrenous in the glands [65]. Usually, mastitis occurs followed by the weakening of the immune system that can happen because of stress or malnutrition [66]. Also, nipple injury is a very predisposal factor. The disease can be both systemic and chronic [67].

CONSENT FOR PUBLICATION

Not applicable.

CONFLICT OF INTEREST

The authors declare no conflict of interest, financial or otherwise.

ACKNOWLEDGEMENTS

Declared none.

REFERENCES

[1]   Turner KH, Everett J, Trivedi U, Rumbaugh KP, Whiteley M. Requirements for *Pseudomonas aeruginosa* acute burn and chronic surgical wound infection. PLoS Genet 2014; 10(7): e1004518.
[http://dx.doi.org/10.1371/journal.pgen.1004518] [PMID: 25057820]

[2]   Driscoll JA, Brody SL, Kollef MH. The epidemiology, pathogenesis and treatment of *Pseudomonas aeruginosa* infections. Drugs 2007; 67(3): 351-68.
[http://dx.doi.org/10.2165/00003495-200767030-00003] [PMID: 17335295]

[3]   Kurahashi K, Kajikawa O, Sawa T, *et al.* Pathogenesis of septic shock in *Pseudomonas aeruginosa* pneumonia. J Clin Invest 1999; 104(6): 743-50.
[http://dx.doi.org/10.1172/JCI7124] [PMID: 10491409]

[4]   Pier GB, Ames P. Mediation of the killing of rough, mucoid isolates of *Pseudomonas aeruginosa* from patients with cystic fibrosis by the alternative pathway of complement. J Infect Dis 1984; 150(2): 223-8.
[http://dx.doi.org/10.1093/infdis/150.2.223] [PMID: 6432921]

[5]   Amiel E, Lovewell RR, O'Toole GA, Hogan DA, Berwin B. *Pseudomonas aeruginosa* evasion of phagocytosis is mediated by loss of swimming motility and is independent of flagellum expression. Infect Immun 2010; 78(7): 2937-45.
[http://dx.doi.org/10.1128/IAI.00144-10] [PMID: 20457788]

[6]   Vaiman M, Lazarovitch T, Heller L, Lotan G. Ecthyma gangrenosum and ecthyma-like lesions: review article. Eur J Clin Microbiol Infect Dis 2015; 34(4): 633-9.
[http://dx.doi.org/10.1007/s10096-014-2277-6] [PMID: 25407372]

[7]   Greene SL, Su WP, Muller SA. Ecthyma gangrenosum: report of clinical, histopathologic, and bacteriologic aspects of eight cases. J Am Acad Dermatol 1984; 11(5 Pt 1): 781-7.
[http://dx.doi.org/10.1016/S0190-9622(84)80453-3] [PMID: 6439763]

[8]   Brown KL, Stein A, Morrell DS. Ecthyma gangrenosum and septic shock syndrome secondary to Chromobacterium violaceum. J Am Acad Dermatol 2006; 54(5) (Suppl.): S224-8.
[http://dx.doi.org/10.1016/j.jaad.2005.07.016] [PMID: 16631946]

[9]   Fink M, Conrad D, Matthews M, Browning JC. Primary ecthyma gangrenosum as a presenting sign of leukemia in a child. Dermatol Online J 2012; 18(3): 3.
[PMID: 22483514]

[10]   Baltch AL, Franke M, Smith RP, *et al.* Serum antibody concentrations of cytotoxin, exotoxin, A, lipopolysaccharide, protease, and elastase and survival of patients with *Pseudomonas aeruginosa* bacteremia. Clin Infect Dis 1996; 23(5): 1109-16.
[http://dx.doi.org/10.1093/clinids/23.5.1109] [PMID: 8922810]

[11]   Pier GB. Pseudomonas and related gram-negative bacillary infections. Goldman's Cecil Medicine 2012; 1877-81.

[12]   Bodey GP, Bolivar R, Fainstein V, Jadeja L. Infections caused by *Pseudomonas aeruginosa*. Rev Infect Dis 1983; 5(2): 279-313.
[http://dx.doi.org/10.1093/clinids/5.2.279] [PMID: 6405475]

[13]   Geraghty T, LaPorta G. Current health and economic burden of chronic diabetic osteomyelitis. Expert Rev Pharmacoecon Outcomes Res 2019; 19(3): 279-86.
[http://dx.doi.org/10.1080/14737167.2019.1567337] [PMID: 30625012]

[14]   Kaya İ, Sezgin B, Eraslan S, Öztürk K, Göde S, Bilgen C, *et al.* Malignant otitis externa: a retrospective analysis and treatment outcomes. Turkish Archives of Otorhinolaryngology 2018; 56(2): 106.

[15]   Gjerde H, Mishra A. Contact lens–related *Pseudomonas aeruginosa* keratitis in a 49-year-old woman. CMAJ 2018; 190(2): E54-E.

[16]   Zimmerman AB, Nixon AD, Rueff EM. Contact lens associated microbial keratitis: practical considerations for the optometrist. Clinical optometry 2016; 8: 1.
[http://dx.doi.org/10.2147/OPTO.S66424]

[17]   Capek KD, Culnan DM, Merkley K, Huang TT, Trocme S. Burn Injuries of the Eye. Total Burn Care. Elsevier 2018; pp. 435-4.
[http://dx.doi.org/10.1016/B978-0-323-47661-4.00041-1]

[18]   Luemsamran P, Pornpanich K, Vangveeravong S, Mekanandha P. Orbital cellulitis and endophthalmitis in pseudomonas septicemia. Orbit 2008; 27(6): 455-7.
[http://dx.doi.org/10.1080/01676830802350422] [PMID: 19085303]

[19]   Ellenberger C, Sturgill BC. Endogenous Pseudomonas Panophthalmitis: Following Prostatic Resection. Am J Ophthalmol 1968; 65(4): 607-11.
[http://dx.doi.org/10.1016/0002-9394(68)93884-1] [PMID: 4966810]

[20]   Ramírez-Estrada S, Borgatta B, Rello J. *Pseudomonas aeruginosa* ventilator-associated pneumonia management. Infect Drug Resist 2016; 9: 7-18.
[PMID: 26855594]

[21]   Obritsch MD, Fish DN, MacLaren R, Jung R. Nosocomial infections due to multidrug-resistant *Pseudomonas aeruginosa*: epidemiology and treatment options. Pharmacotherapy 2005; 25(10): 1353-64.
[http://dx.doi.org/10.1592/phco.2005.25.10.1353] [PMID: 16185180]

[22]   Li Z, Kosorok MR, Farrell PM, *et al.* Longitudinal development of mucoid *Pseudomonas aeruginosa* infection and lung disease progression in children with cystic fibrosis. JAMA 2005; 293(5): 581-8.
[http://dx.doi.org/10.1001/jama.293.5.581] [PMID: 15687313]

[23]   Warren AE, Boulianne-Larsen CM, Chandler CB, *et al.* Genotypic and phenotypic variation in *Pseudomonas aeruginosa* reveals signatures of secondary infection and mutator activity in certain cystic fibrosis patients with chronic lung infections. Infect Immun 2011; 79(12): 4802-18.
[http://dx.doi.org/10.1128/IAI.05282-11] [PMID: 21930755]

[24]   Evans SE, Ost DE. Pneumonia in the neutropenic cancer patient. Curr Opin Pulm Med 2015; 21(3): 260-71.
[http://dx.doi.org/10.1097/MCP.0000000000000156] [PMID: 25784246]

[25]   Moghaddam SJ, Ochoa CE, Sethi S, Dickey BF. Nontypeable Haemophilus influenzae in chronic obstructive pulmonary disease and lung cancer. Int J Chron Obstruct Pulmon Dis 2011; 6: 113-23.
[http://dx.doi.org/10.2147/COPD.S15417] [PMID: 21407824]

[26]   Defres S, Marwick C, Nathwani D. MRSA as a cause of lung infection including airway infection, community-acquired pneumonia and hospital-acquired pneumonia. Eur Respir J 2009; 34(6): 1470-6.
[http://dx.doi.org/10.1183/09031936.00122309] [PMID: 19948913]

[27]   Schweizer F, Jiao H, Hindsgaul O, Wong WY, Irvin RT. Interaction between the pili of *Pseudomonas aeruginosa* PAK and its carbohydrate receptor β-D-GalNAc(1-->4)β-D-Gal analogs. Can J Microbiol 1998; 44(3): 307-11.
[PMID: 9606914]

[28]   Riquelme SA, Hopkins BD, Wolfe AL, DiMango E, Kitur K, Parsons R, *et al.* Cystic fibrosis transmembrane conductance regulator attaches tumor suppressor PTEN to the membrane and promotes anti *Pseudomonas aeruginosa* immunity. Immunity 2017; 47(6): 1169-81.
[http://dx.doi.org/10.1016/j.immuni.2017.11.010]

[29]   Gellatly SL, Hancock RE. *Pseudomonas aeruginosa*: new insights into pathogenesis and host defenses. Pathog Dis 2013; 67(3): 159-73.
[http://dx.doi.org/10.1111/2049-632X.12033] [PMID: 23620179]

[30]   Tohyama M. CFTR as cAMP-dependent chloride channels and as cAMP-dependent regulator of sodium channels. Nihon Rinsho 1996; 54(2): 429-33.
[PMID: 8838092]

[31]   Poletti V, Casoni G, Chilosi M, Zompatori M. Diffuse panbronchiolitis. Eur Respir J 2006; 28(4): 862-71.
[http://dx.doi.org/10.1183/09031936.06.00131805] [PMID: 17012632]

[32]   Keicho N, Kudoh S. Diffuse panbronchiolitis: role of macrolides in therapy. Am J Respir Med 2002; 1(2): 119-31.
[http://dx.doi.org/10.1007/BF03256601] [PMID: 14720066]

[33]   Lamas Ferreiro JL, Álvarez Otero J, González González L, *et al. Pseudomonas aeruginosa* urinary tract infections in hospitalized patients: Mortality and prognostic factors. PLoS One 2017; 12(5): e0178178.
[http://dx.doi.org/10.1371/journal.pone.0178178] [PMID: 28552972]

[34]   Chang SL, Shortliffe LD. Pediatric urinary tract infections. Pediatr Clin North Am 2006; 53(3): 379-400.
[http://dx.doi.org/10.1016/j.pcl.2006.02.011] [PMID: 16716786]

[35]   Kucheria R, Dasgupta P, Sacks SH, Khan MS, Sheerin NS. Urinary tract infections: new insights into a common problem. Postgrad Med J 2005; 81(952): 83-6.
[http://dx.doi.org/10.1136/pgmj.2004.023036] [PMID: 15701738]

[36]   Williams D, Schaeffer AJ. Current concepts in urinary tract infections. Minerva urologica e nefrologica Italian J Urol Nephrol 2004; 56(1): 15-31.

[37]   Bonadio M, Meini M, Gigli C, Longo B, Vigna A. Urinary tract infection in diabetic patients. Urol Int 1999; 63(4): 215-9.
[http://dx.doi.org/10.1159/000030453] [PMID: 10743697]

[38]   Warren JW, Tenney JH, Hoopes JM, Muncie HL, Anthony WC. A prospective microbiologic study of bacteriuria in patients with chronic indwelling urethral catheters. J Infect Dis 1982; 146(6): 719-23.
[http://dx.doi.org/10.1093/infdis/146.6.719] [PMID: 6815281]

[39]   Mittal R, Aggarwal S, Sharma S, Chhibber S, Harjai K. Urinary tract infections caused by *Pseudomonas aeruginosa*: a minireview. J Infect Public Health 2009; 2(3): 101-11.
[http://dx.doi.org/10.1016/j.jiph.2009.08.003] [PMID: 20701869]

[40]   Norbury W, Herndon DN, Tanksley J, Jeschke MG, Finnerty CC. Infection in Burns. Surg Infect (Larchmt) 2016; 17(2): 250-5.
[http://dx.doi.org/10.1089/sur.2013.134] [PMID: 26978531]

[41]   Wu DC, Chan WW, Metelitsa AI, Fiorillo L, Lin AN. Pseudomonas skin infection: clinical features, epidemiology, and management. Am J Clin Dermatol 2011; 12(3): 157-69.
[http://dx.doi.org/10.2165/11539770-000000000-00000] [PMID: 21469761]

[42]   Holzheimer RG, Mannick JA. Surgical treatment: evidence-based and problem-oriented: Zuckschwerdt 2001.

[43]   Yu Y, Cheng AS, Wang L, Dunne WM, Bayliss SJ. Hot tub folliculitis or hot hand-foot syndrome caused by *Pseudomonas aeruginosa*. J Am Acad Dermatol 2007; 57(4): 596-600.

[http://dx.doi.org/10.1016/j.jaad.2007.04.004] [PMID: 17658195]

[44] Abramson C. Athlete's foot caused by *Pseudomonas aeruginosa*. Clin Dermatol 1983; 1(1): 14-24.
[http://dx.doi.org/10.1016/0738-081X(83)90037-8] [PMID: 6443779]

[45] Nenoff P, Paasch U, Handrick W. Infections of finger and toe nails due to fungi and bacteria. Der Hautarzt; Zeitschrift fur Dermatologie, Venerologie, und verwandte Gebiete 2014; 65(4): 337-48.

[46] Müller S, Ebnöther M, Itin P. Green nail syndrome (*Pseudomonas aeruginosa* nail infection): two cases successfully treated with topical nadifloxacin, an acne medication. Case Rep Dermatol 2014; 6(2): 180-4.
[http://dx.doi.org/10.1159/000365863] [PMID: 25202260]

[47] Gul S, Eraj A, Ashraf Z. *Pseudomonas aeruginosa*: A common causative agent of ear infections in South Asian children. Int J Curr Microbiol Appl Sci 2014; 3: 156-60.

[48] Morris P. Chronic suppurative otitis media. BMJ clinical evidence 2012.

[49] Selimoglu E. Aminoglycoside-induced ototoxicity. Curr Pharm Des 2007; 13(1): 119-26.
[http://dx.doi.org/10.2174/138161207779313731] [PMID: 17266591]

[50] Wieland M, Lederman MM, Kline-King C, *et al*. Left-sided endocarditis due to *Pseudomonas aeruginosa*. A report of 10 cases and review of the literature. Medicine (Baltimore) 1986; 65(3): 180-9.
[http://dx.doi.org/10.1097/00005792-198605000-00006] [PMID: 3084905]

[51] Dawson NL, Brumble LM, Pritt BS, Yao JD, Echols JD, Alvarez S. Left-sided *Pseudomonas aeruginosa* endocarditis in patients without injection drug use. Medicine (Baltimore) 2011; 90(4): 250-5.
[http://dx.doi.org/10.1097/MD.0b013e3182252133] [PMID: 21694647]

[52] Sousa C, Botelho C, Rodrigues D, Azeredo J, Oliveira R. Infective endocarditis in intravenous drug abusers: an update. Eur J Clin Microbiol Infect Dis 2012; 31(11): 2905-10.
[http://dx.doi.org/10.1007/s10096-012-1675-x] [PMID: 22714640]

[53] Cahill TJ, Baddour LM, Habib G, *et al*. Challenges in infective endocarditis. J Am Coll Cardiol 2017; 69(3): 325-44.
[http://dx.doi.org/10.1016/j.jacc.2016.10.066] [PMID: 28104075]

[54] Saraiva RM, Camillis LF, Francisco RM, Gomes MV. Isolated pulmonary valve *Pseudomonas aeruginosa* endocarditis related to catheter embolism. Int J Cardiol 2002; 83(1): 83-4.
[http://dx.doi.org/10.1016/S0167-5273(01)00613-1] [PMID: 11959388]

[55] Ramadan FB, Beanlands DS, Burwash IG. Isolated pulmonic valve endocarditis in healthy hearts: a case report and review of the literature. Can J Cardiol 2000; 16(10): 1282-8.
[PMID: 11064303]

[56] Pomar V, Benito N, López-Contreras J, Coll P, Gurguí M, Domingo P. Spontaneous gram-negative bacillary meningitis in adult patients: characteristics and outcome. BMC Infect Dis 2013; 13(1): 451.
[http://dx.doi.org/10.1186/1471-2334-13-451] [PMID: 24079517]

[57] Gupta SK, Rana AS, Gupta D, Jain G, Kalra P. Unusual causes of reduced mouth opening and it's suitable surgical management: Our experience. Natl J Maxillofac Surg 2010; 1(1): 86-90.
[http://dx.doi.org/10.4103/0975-5950.69150] [PMID: 22442560]

[58] Komshian SV, Tablan OC, Palutke W, Reyes MP. Characteristics of left-sided endocarditis due to *Pseudomonas aeruginosa* in the Detroit Medical Center. Rev Infect Dis 1990; 12(4): 693-702.
[http://dx.doi.org/10.1093/clinids/12.4.693] [PMID: 2385771]

[59] Greenlee JE. Subdural Empyema. Curr Treat Options Neurol 2003; 5(1): 13-22.
[http://dx.doi.org/10.1007/s11940-003-0019-7] [PMID: 12521560]

[60] Nussbaum ES, Rigamonti D, Standiford H, Numaguchi Y, Wolf AL, Robinson WL. Spinal epidural abscess: a report of 40 cases and review. Surg Neurol 1992; 38(3): 225-31.

[http://dx.doi.org/10.1016/0090-3019(92)90173-K] [PMID: 1359657]

[61]   Dold H. On pyocyaneus sepsis and intestinal infections in Shanghai due to *Bacillus pyocyaneus*. Chin Med J (Engl) 1918; 32: 435.

[62]   Spencer LV, Callen JP. Cutaneous manifestations of bacterial infections. Dermatol Clin 1989; 7(3): 579-89.
        [http://dx.doi.org/10.1016/S0733-8635(18)30587-4] [PMID: 2665988]

[63]   Halder P, Mandal KC, Mukhopadhyay M, Debnath B. Shanghai fever: a fatal form of *Pseudomonas aeruginosa* enteric disease. Indian Pediatr 2015; 52(10): 896-8.
        [http://dx.doi.org/10.1007/s13312-015-0741-8] [PMID: 26499020]

[64]   Meretoja T, Ihalainen H, Leidenius M. Inflammations of the mammary gland. Duodecim; laaketieteellinen aikakauskirja 2017; 133(9): 855-61.

[65]   Kelly EJ, Wilson DJ. *Pseudomonas aeruginosa* mastitis in two goats associated with an essential oil-based teat dip. J Vet Diagn Invest 2016; 28(6): 760-2.
        [http://dx.doi.org/10.1177/1040638716672255] [PMID: 27698173]

[66]   Kirk JH, Bartlett PC. Nonclinical *Pseudomonas aeruginosa* mastitis in a dairy herd. J Am Vet Med Assoc 1984; 184(6): 671-3.
        [PMID: 6427159]

[67]   Baron S. Alphaviruses (Togaviridae) and Flaviviruses (Flaviviridae)--Medical Microbiology: University of Texas Medical Branch at Galveston 1996.

CHAPTER 6

Laboratory Diagnosis

M. Mahmoudi[1], S. Ghafourian[1,*], H. Kazemian[1] and **B. Badaksh[2]**

[1] *Department of Microbiology, Faculty of Medicine, Ilam University of Medical Sciences, Ilam, Iran*

[2] *Department of Gastroenterology, Faculty of Medicine, Ilam University of Medical Sciences, Ilam, Iran*

Abstract: Due to the high potency of *P. aeruginosa* in pathogenesis and diffusion in the human body, it can be diagnosed in a variety of clinical specimens. For this purpose, the unique properties of *P. aeruginosa* are used. In general, the appearance of the bacterium under the microscope and its features on culture media as well as biochemical tests are widely used for the initial diagnosis of *P. aeruginosa* in the clinical laboratories. In this section, the diagnostic routine tests are briefly discussed so the readers can easily use them.

Keywords: Gram-negative bacteria, Phenotypic identification.

P. aeruginosa could be isolated from a variety of specimens based on the type of the infection including, blood, urine, sputum, spinal fluid, pus, skin injured tissues [1].

P. aeruginosa is a rod shape gram-negative bacteria, which measures 0.5 to 0.8 µm by 1.5 to 3.0 µm. Both the catalase and oxidase tests are positive [2].The result of the culture in the Kligler's Iron Agar (KIA) is alk/alk after 18-24hr at 35°C [3]. As well, the negative results are observed for using glucose, production of H^2S and gas [4].

Also, weak positive motility can be seen [5]. In addition, *P. aeruginosa* isolates are beta-hemolytic on blood agar [6]. It can grow on cetrimide agar and usually produce blue-green color pigments that name pyocyanin (king A agar is specific media for detection of the pigments). It can also grows at 42°C, which can be used to distinguish it from many other *Pseudomonas* species (Fig. **1**) [7].

* **Corresponding author S. Ghafourian:** Department of Microbiology, Faculty of Medicine, Ilam University of Medical Sciences, Iran; E-mail: sobhan.ghafurian@gmail.com

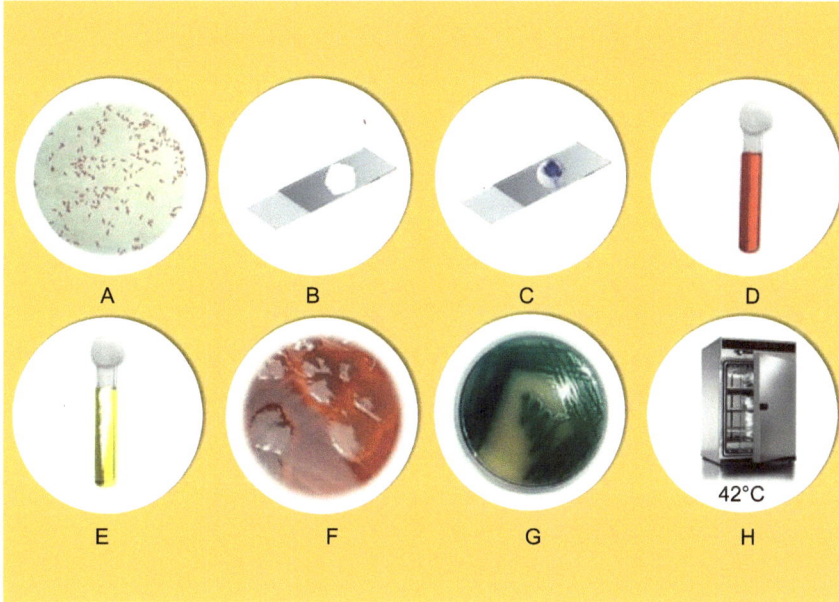

Fig. (1). Laboratory diagnosis of *P. aeruginosa*. **(A)** Gram staining. *P. aeruginosa* is gram-negative bacteria, which appears as rods under the microscope. **(B)** Catalase test. It is catalase-positive, which is determined by the observation of oxygen bubbles when hydrogen peroxide is added to the bacterium. **(C)** Oxidase test. It is oxidase-positive, which can be observed by the production of purple color on oxidase disk by adding a loop of the bacterium and a small amount of distilled water. **(D)** Grows on Kligler's Iron Agar: the result is alk/alk after 18-24 hr at 35°C. **(E)** Grows on SIM (Sulfur, Indole, Motility): it is motile, which can be detected by creating turbidity in the culture line. **(F)** analysis of hemolysis on blood agar: It causes complete lysis of red blood cells, which is seen as a transparent halo around the colonies. **(G)** Grows on cetrimide agar: cetrimide used as a detergent to selects *P. aeruginosa* from alternate microbial flora. It also produces a significant amount of pyocyanin, which is a blue-green color. **(H)** Grows at 42°C: *P. aeruginosa* grows uniquely at 42°C. This specific temperature isolates *P. aeruginosa* from non-pigmented *P. aeruginosa* and the other species of fluorescent pseudomonads.

CONSENT FOR PUBLICATION

Not applicable.

CONFLICT OF INTEREST

The authors declare no conflict of interest, financial or otherwise.

ACKNOWLEDGEMENTS

Declared none.

REFERENCES

[1]   Carroll KC, Butel J, Morse S. Jawetz Melnick and Adelbergs Medical Microbiology 27 E. McGraw-Hill Education 2015.

[2]   Baron S. Alphaviruses (Togaviridae) and Flaviviruses (Flaviviridae)--Medical Microbiology. Galveston: University of Texas Medical Branch 1996.

[3]   Hashim IA, Wdaah QH, Atya AA. Potential effect of antimicrobial agents against *Staphylococcus aureus* and *Pseudomonas aeruginosa* strains from patients with skin infections. Uni Thi-Qar J Sci 2019; 7(1): 7-14.

[4]   Banerjee S, Batabyal K, Joardar SN, *et al.* Detection and characterization of pathogenic *Pseudomonas aeruginosa* from bovine subclinical mastitis in West Bengal, India. Vet World 2017; 10(7): 738-42.
[http://dx.doi.org/10.14202/vetworld.2017.738-742] [PMID: 28831214]

[5]   Luzar MA, Thomassen MJ, Montie TC. Flagella and motility alterations in *Pseudomonas aeruginosa* strains from patients with cystic fibrosis: relationship to patient clinical condition. Infect Immun 1985; 50(2): 577-82.
[http://dx.doi.org/10.1128/IAI.50.2.577-582.1985] [PMID: 3932214]

[6]   Reyes EA, Bale MJ, Cannon WH, Matsen JM. Identification of *Pseudomonas aeruginosa* by pyocyanin production on Tech agar. J Clin Microbiol 1981; 13(3): 456-8.
[http://dx.doi.org/10.1128/JCM.13.3.456-458.1981] [PMID: 6787067]

[7]   Brown VI, Lowbury EJ. Use of an improved cetrimide agar medium and other culture methods for *Pseudomonas aeruginosa*. J Clin Pathol 1965; 18(6): 752-6.
[http://dx.doi.org/10.1136/jcp.18.6.752] [PMID: 4954265]

CHAPTER 7

Antibiotic Resistance and Treatment

M. Mahmoudi[1], S. Ghafourian[1,*], H. Kazemian[1] and B. Badakhsh[2]

[1] *Department of Microbiology, Faculty of Medicine, Ilam University of Medical Sciences, Ilam, Iran*

[2] *Department of Gastroenterology, Faculty of Medicine, Ilam University of Medical Sciences, Ilam*

Abstract: *P. aeruginosa* belongs to the group of the pathogens that is in dire need of the novel and effective drugs. Meanwhile, carbapenem-resistant *P. aeruginosa* strains located at the first line of the emergency. Currently, both monotherapy and combination therapy are used for the treatment, but they are not always effective. One of the major reasons for the failure of treatment is the severe antibiotic resistance of *P. aeruginosa*. In addition to the inherent antibiotic resistance of this bacterium, it can also receive the antibiotic resistance gene from its environment. Also, the role of genetic mutations and improper use of antibiotics should not be underestimated in these kinds of resistances. There is another considerable point about antibiotic resistance of *P. aeruginosa*, which is its ability to the formation of recalcitrant biofilm and persister cells. Over time, several antibiotics have been used to treat *P. aeruginosa*, but unfortunately, they have lost their healing power one after another. Penicillin, aminoglycosides, third generation of cephalosporin are examples of these antibiotics. Imipenem and meropenem are currently being used to treat *P. aeruginosa* severe infections. But, resistance to both of them is also increasing. Unfortunately, many *P. aeruginosa* strains have also been identified that are resistant to all available antibiotics. Nevertheless, researchers are trying to find new drugs and they have partly succeeded. Some newly introduced antibiotics include plazomicin, doripenem, and POL7001. Anyway, we still need novel and more effective drugs against *P. aeruginosa* infections.

Keywords: β-lactam antibiotics, Aminoglycosides, Biofilm, Carbapenems, Combination therapy, Doripenem, Efflux pump, ESBLs, PER, Persister cell, Plazomicin, POL7001 pandrug resistance isolates, Third generation cephalosporins, VIM.

---

* **Corresponding author S. Ghafourian:** Department of Microbiology, Faculty of Medicine, Ilam University of Medical Sciences, Iran; E-mail: sobhan.ghafurian@gmail.com

Mina Mahmoudi, Sobhan Ghafourian & Behzad Badakhsh (Eds.)

In 2017, the World Health Organization (WHO) published the list of bacteria, which urgently need new antibiotics. Among this list, the *P. aeruginosa*, carbapenem-resistant allocated the second rank to itself [1]. Hence, in the view of some, just this one point is sufficient to prove the necessity of research and investigation on *P. aeruginosa* in all dimensions.

Nevertheless, monotherapy and combination therapy are still used but it doesn't work for all cases [2]. *P. aeruginosa* has different and powerful mechanisms to counteract with the antibiotics. Firstly, it has intrinsic antibiotic resistance. For instance, using efflux pumps is one of the effective ways to combat antibiotics. Efflux pumps sending out the antibiotics that have been seceded to enter into *P. aeruginosa* [3]. The other one is the low capacity of the outer membrane to pass the antibiotic through itself. So, many antibiotics cannot even enter into *P. aeruginosa*. For example, there are a variety of antibiotics that their desired targets are located inside the bacterial cell including aminoglycosides, polymyxins, quinolones, and β-lactams. Based on this ability of *P. aeruginosa*, these antibiotics faced with a challenge to reach their desired targets. In addition, *P. aeruginosa* is able to produce specific enzymes that can inactivate antibiotics.

Sometimes *P. aeruginosa* adapts itself to survive in the presence of antibiotics. For instance, as the lungs of cystic fibrosis patients are very favorable for the *P. aeruginosa*, it can easily form the biofilm and escape from the antibiotics. As well, sometimes the biofilm contains very specific cells named persister [4]. The persister cells are dormant and form by the unclear pathways that are incredibly persisting against antibiotics. Some literature claimed that persister cells could not be killed even by 1000 fold antibiotics concentrations [5].

Lastly, *P. aeruginosa* can acquire resistance genes from the environment, which occur by horizontal transform of the antibiotic resistance genes. As well, mutations can also contribute to the appearance of antibiotic resistance (Fig. **1**) [6].

Here is an overview of the history of antibiotic resistance in *P. aeruginosa* during the time. Like many other organisms, penicillin was also used for the treatment of *P. aeruginosa*. But due to the high ability of *P. aeruginosa* to adapt to environmental stimuli, many strains became resistant to penicillin [7]. Based on this, physicians started to prescribe aminoglycosides such as streptomycin, kanamycin, and tobramycin [8]. But, unfortunately, still resistance to aminoglycosides, like the flow of a roaring river, encompassed most of the strains. The next weapon was the third generation of cephalosporin including, ceftazidime, cefotaxime and ceftriaxone [9]. Not too long after that this weapon also failed to struggle with *P. aeruginosa* [8]. At this time, scientists recommended to prescribe aminoglycosides in combination with the third generation of the cephalosporin. For instance, they used the combination of ceftazidime with tobramycin (Fig. **1**) [10].

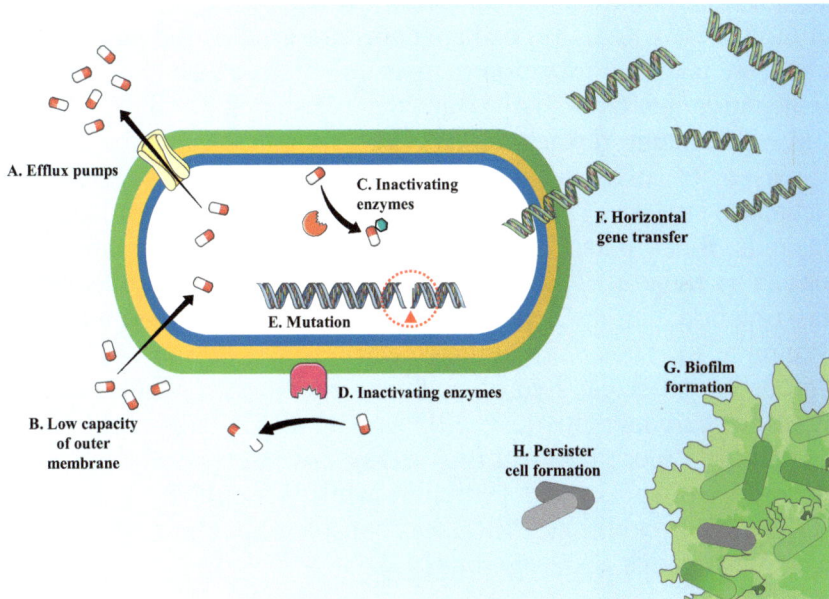

Fig. (1). Mechanisms of antibiotic resistance in *P. aeruginosa*. **(A)** Efflux pumps: efflux pumps are transport antibiotics from within cells into the external environment and cause multidrug resistance in *P. aeruginosa*. **(B)** low capacity of outer membrane: several *P. aeruginosa* antibiotics targets are located inside of the cell. So, antibiotics must entire into the cell and reach their targets. Low capacity of the outer membrane contracts with this event by standing against antibiotics as a barrier. **(C and D)** Inactivating enzymes: inactivating enzymes interact with antibiotics and inactivate them against bacteria. beta-lactamase enzymes are the most popular inactivating enzymes against beta-lactam antibiotics including, penicillins, and cephalosporins. **(E)** Mutation: In some cases, random mutations that occur naturally in the bacterial population can cause antibiotic resistance. **(F)** Horizontal gene transfer (HGT): genetic materials transfer between strains and species through HGT. Sometimes these genetic materials carry antibiotic resistance genes that spread through the bacterial population by multiple mechanisms. **(G)** Biofilm formation: *P. aeruginosa* forms the strongest bacterial biofilm, which can be introduced as the most important factor in antibiotic resistance. Biofilm contracts with antibiotics through several mechanisms. In summary, it acts as a barrier and prevents the penetration of antibiotics in to the depth of the biofilm. In addition, neutralizing enzymes are presented in higher concentrations in biofilm and as soon as the antibiotics penetrate, they neutralize them. Some biofilm structural materials also trap antibiotics. **(H)** Persister cell formation: Persister cells are dormant cells that are tolerant against antibiotics. *P. aeruginosa* persister cells have been reported in biofilm, which is very important in the treatment and infection control of patients with cystic fibrosis.

Subsequently, due to the resistance to third generation of the cephalosporin, new strains were emerged named extended spectrum beta-lactamase [11]. These strains produced high levels of antibacterial enzymes that caused severe antibiotic resistance.

Given the dramatic pace of antibiotic resistance, the last choice left for the physicians was describing the imipenem and meropenem [12]. Imipenem and meropenem are both members of carbapenems, which belongs to the class of beta-lactam antibiotics [13]. Usually, carbapenems are used as the last choice in the treatment of severe bacterial infection such as infections caused by multidrug-resistant Gram-negative bacteria [14]. But, the resistance to imipenem and meropenem is also increasing devastatingly [15]. Production of carbapenemase enzymes is the reason for resistance, which included serine carbapenemase and metallo-beta-lactamase enzymes [16]. Carbapenemase encoding genes are usually encoded on plasmids. Since plasmids are mobile genetic elements, carbapenem resistance genes can spread quickly in the bacterial populations [17]. According to the Ambler Classification, carbapenem-hydrolyzing enzymes divided into the A, B, C, and D groups [18]. Hence, extended-spectrum beta-lactamases (ESBLs) belongs to the group A, which can hydrolyze third-generation cephalosporins and monobactams but not carbapenems [19, 20]. Among ESBL enzymes,PER and VEB enzymes are mostly more frequent in *P. aeruginosa* [21]. PER-1 enzyme is able to hydrolyze cephalosporin and penicillin while it could be inhibited by clavulanic acid [22, 23]. In addition, PER-1 has considerable clinical importance due to the high activity against *P. aeruginosa* [24].

Subsequently, group B was divided into the three subgroups BI, BII, and BIII. BI classified into the four groups based on their molecular structure including IPM, SPM, VIM, and GIM [25]. Currently, VIM (Verona integron-encoded metallo -β -lactamase) is the most widespread type of *P. aeruginosa* around the world. VIM-positive *P. aeruginosa* is able to cause nosocomial infections and it is responsible for multiple outbreaks [26]. Laboratory diagnosis of VIM and PER consists of antibiogram, E-test (Epsilometer test) and detection of bela VIM and bla PER, MBL and ESBL genes by PCR [21, 27]. Besides, a *P. aeruginosa* strain was reported from Italy that harbored both PER-1 and VIM-2 together. In other words, this microorganism is resistant to all antibiotics [28].

Totally, there are *P. aeruginosa* strains, which are resistant to all commercially available antibiotics. So that, these strains showed antibiotic resistance to penicillin, ceftazidime, cephalosporins, aztreonam, carbapenems, amino glycosides, and ciprofloxacin, and so-called pandrug-resistance isolates [29]. In fact, *P. aeruginosa* is resistant to most antimicrobial agents.

Recently, some antibiotics are recommended for the treatment of *P. aeruginosa* that they have other modes of action comparing with the previous medicines. Although new antibiotics are much more effective, they also show lower levels of resistance [4]. A number of these novel antibiotics are, plazomicin, doripenem, and POL7001 [30].

Plazomicin demonstrated antibacterial effect to both Gram-negative and Gram-positive bacteria in the *in vitro* condition. In addition, the mode of action of plazomicin has resembled to amikacin [31]. Plazomicin is a semisynthetic aminoglycoside that is derived from sisomicin (Ensamysin). In addition, it was isolated from *Micromonospora inyoensis* species [32, 33]. Nevertheless, there is a negative tip about plazomicin, which is an intermediate nephrotoxic activity [34].

Doripenem also is one of the newly carbapenem antibiotics and it is also effective against both gram positive and Gram-negative bacteria. Several β-lactamases cannot hydrolyze doripenem [35, 36].

Another protein epitope mimetic antibiotic showed nicely effect against *P. aeruginosa* named POL7001. This antibiotic acts against transportation of the LPS to outer membrane [37].

Although some antibiotics are empirically prescribed for treatment of *P. aeruginosa* but bacterial resistance pattern is also strongly correlated with geographical area and health status of the region [38]. Accordingly, it is highly suggested that once the empirical treatment is started, the determination of antibiotic susceptibility of isolates also should be started. The necessity of this issue will be very pressing when the experimental treatment fails, because at this crucial moment, possessing a second treatment can save the life of the severe patients. Subsequently, empirical treatments are also associated with the type of infections [39]. In addition, *P. aeruginosa* utilizes different strategies to escape treatment. For this reason, monotherapy fails in most cases and combination therapy has much more popularity [30]. Generally, drugs used against *P. aeruginosa* are aztreonam, carbapenems (meropenem and imipenem) and fluoroquinolones (ciprofloxacin), cephalosporins (ceftazidime, cefoperazone, andcefepime) [40, 41]. As well, for the combination therapy, an extended-spectrum penicillin is used with an aminoglycoside. For instance, the combination of piperacillin with tobramycin is common [42].

CONSENT FOR PUBLICATION

Not applicable.

CONFLICT OF INTEREST

The authors declare no conflict of interest, financial or otherwise.

ACKNOWLEDGEMENTS

Declared none.

REFERENCES

[1]   Wieland M, Lederman MM, Kline-King C, *et al.* Left-sided endocarditis due to *Pseudomonas aeruginosa*. A report of 10 cases and review of the literature. Medicine (Baltimore) 1986; 65(3): 180-9.
[http://dx.doi.org/10.1097/00005792-198605000-00006] [PMID: 3084905]

[2]   El Solh AA, Alhajhusain A. Update on the treatment of *Pseudomonas aeruginosa* pneumonia. J Antimicrob Chemother 2009; 64(2): 229-38.
[http://dx.doi.org/10.1093/jac/dkp201] [PMID: 19520717]

[3]   Aeschlimann JR. Insights from the Society of Infectious Diseases Pharmacists. The role of multidrug efflux pumps in the antibiotic resistance of *Pseudomonas aeruginosa* and other gram-negative bacteria. Pharmacotherapy 2003; 23(7): 916-24.
[http://dx.doi.org/10.1592/phco.23.7.916.32722] [PMID: 12885104]

[4]   Chatterjee M, Anju CP, Biswas L, Anil Kumar V, Gopi Mohan C, Biswas R. Antibiotic resistance in *Pseudomonas aeruginosa* and alternative therapeutic options. Int J Med Microbiol 2016; 306(1): 48-58.
[http://dx.doi.org/10.1016/j.ijmm.2015.11.004] [PMID: 26687205]

[5]   Maisonneuve E, Gerdes K. Molecular mechanisms underlying bacterial persisters. Cell 2014; 157(3): 539-48.
[http://dx.doi.org/10.1016/j.cell.2014.02.050] [PMID: 24766804]

[6]   Lambert PA. Mechanisms of antibiotic resistance in *Pseudomonas aeruginosa*. J R Soc Med 2002; 95 (Suppl. 41): 22-6.
[PMID: 12216271]

[7]   Wolter DJ, Lister PD. Mechanisms of β-lactam resistance among *Pseudomonas aeruginosa*. Curr Pharm Des 2013; 19(2): 209-22.
[http://dx.doi.org/10.2174/138161213804070311] [PMID: 22894618]

[8]   Clark RB, Sanders CC, Pakiz CB, Hostetter MK. Aminoglycoside resistance among *Pseudomonas aeruginosa* isolates with an unusual disk diffusion antibiogram. Antimicrob Agents Chemother 1988; 32(5): 689-92.
[http://dx.doi.org/10.1128/AAC.32.5.689] [PMID: 3134846]

[9]   Puri J, Revathi G, Kundra P, Talwar V. Activity of third generation cephalosporins against *Pseudomonas aeruginosa* in high risk hospital units. Indian J Med Sci 1996; 50(7): 239-43.
[PMID: 8979542]

[10]   Mayer I, Nagy E. Investigation of the synergic effects of aminoglycoside-fluoroquinolone and third-generation cephalosporin combinations against clinical isolates of Pseudomonas spp. J Antimicrob Chemother 1999; 43(5): 651-7.
[http://dx.doi.org/10.1093/jac/43.5.651] [PMID: 10382886]

[11]   Blaak H, Lynch G, Italiaander R, Hamidjaja RA, Schets FM, de Roda Husman AM. Multidrug-resistant and extended spectrum beta-lactamase-producing *Escherichia coli* in Dutch surface water and wastewater. PLoS One 2015; 10(6): e0127752.
[http://dx.doi.org/10.1371/journal.pone.0127752] [PMID: 26030904]

[12]   Rodríguez-Martínez J-M, Poirel L, Nordmann P. Molecular epidemiology and mechanisms of carbapenem resistance in *Pseudomonas aeruginosa*. Antimicrob Agents Chemother 2009; 53(11): 4783-8.
[http://dx.doi.org/10.1128/AAC.00574-09] [PMID: 19738025]

[13]   Hellinger WC, Brewer NS. Carbapenems and monobactams: imipenem, meropenem, and aztreonam. Mayo Clin Proc 1999; 74(4): 420-34.
[http://dx.doi.org/10.4065/74.4.420] [PMID: 10221472]

[14]   Elshamy AA, Aboshanab KM. A review on bacterial resistance to carbapenems: epidemiology, detection and treatment options. Future Sci OA 2020; 6(3): FSO438.
[http://dx.doi.org/10.2144/fsoa-2019-0098] [PMID: 32140243]

[15]   Slama TG. Clinical review: balancing the therapeutic, safety, and economic issues underlying effective antipseudomonal carbapenem use. Crit Care 2008; 12(5): 233.
[http://dx.doi.org/10.1186/cc6994] [PMID: 18983709]

[16]   Queenan AM, Bush K. Carbapenemases: the versatile beta-lactamases. Clin Microbiol Rev 2007; 20(3): 440-58.
[http://dx.doi.org/10.1128/CMR.00001-07] [PMID: 17630334]

[17]   Stadler M, Dersch P, Heinz D. How to overcome the antibiotic crisis facts, challenges, technologies and future perspectives preface. Springer-verlag berlin heidelberger platz 3, d-14197 berlin. Germany 2016.
[http://dx.doi.org/10.1007/978-3-319-49284-1]

[18]   Bush K, Jacoby GA. Updated functional classification of β-lactamases. Antimicrob Agents Chemother 2010; 54(3): 969-76.
[http://dx.doi.org/10.1128/AAC.01009-09] [PMID: 19995920]

[19]   Weldhagen GF, Poirel L, Nordmann P. Ambler class A extended-spectrum beta-lactamases in *Pseudomonas aeruginosa*: novel developments and clinical impact. Antimicrob Agents Chemother 2003; 47(8): 2385-92.
[http://dx.doi.org/10.1128/AAC.47.8.2385-2392.2003] [PMID: 12878494]

[20]   Ali T, Ali I, Khan NA, Han B, Gao J. The growing genetic and functional diversity of extended spectrum beta-lactamases. BioMed research international 2018.

[21]   Laudy AE, Róg P, Smolińska-Król K, *et al.* Prevalence of ESBL-producing *Pseudomonas aeruginosa* isolates in Warsaw, Poland, detected by various phenotypic and genotypic methods. PLoS One 2017; 12(6): e0180121.
[http://dx.doi.org/10.1371/journal.pone.0180121] [PMID: 28658322]

[22]   Nordmann P, Naas T. Sequence analysis of PER-1 extended-spectrum beta-lactamase from *Pseudomonas aeruginosa* and comparison with class A beta-lactamases. Antimicrob Agents Chemother 1994; 38(1): 104-14.
[http://dx.doi.org/10.1128/AAC.38.1.104] [PMID: 8141562]

[23]   Nordmann P, Ronco E, Naas T, Duport C, Michel-Briand Y, Labia R. Characterization of a novel extended-spectrum beta-lactamase from *Pseudomonas aeruginosa*. Antimicrob Agents Chemother 1993; 37(5): 962-9.
[http://dx.doi.org/10.1128/AAC.37.5.962] [PMID: 8517722]

[24]   Empel J, Filczak K, Mrówka A, Hryniewicz W, Livermore DM, Gniadkowski M. Outbreak of *Pseudomonas aeruginosa* infections with PER-1 extended-spectrum β-lactamase in Warsaw, Poland: further evidence for an international clonal complex. J Clin Microbiol 2007; 45(9): 2829-34.
[http://dx.doi.org/10.1128/JCM.00997-07] [PMID: 17634312]

[25]   Aghamiri S, Amirmozafari N, Fallah Mehrabadi J, Fouladtan B, Samadi Kafil H. Antibiotic resistance pattern and evaluation of metallo-beta lactamase genes including bla-IMP and bla-VIM types in *Pseudomonas aeruginosa* isolated from patients in Tehran hospitals. International Scholarly Research Notices 2014.

[26]   Hong DJ, Bae IK, Jang I-H, Jeong SH, Kang H-K, Lee K. Epidemiology and characteristics of metallo-β-lactamase-producing *Pseudomonas aeruginosa*. Infect Chemother 2015; 47(2): 81-97.
[http://dx.doi.org/10.3947/ic.2015.47.2.81] [PMID: 26157586]

[27]   El-Ageery SM, Al-Hazmi SS. Microbiological and molecular detection of VIM-1 metallo beta lactamase-producing *Acinetobacter baumannii*. Eur Rev Med Pharmacol Sci 2014; 18(7): 965-70.
[PMID: 24763874]

[28]   Docquier J-D, Luzzaro F, Amicosante G, Toniolo A, Rossolini GM. Multidrug-resistant *Pseudomonas aeruginosa* producing PER-1 extended-spectrum serine-beta-lactamase and VIM-2 metallo-bet--lactamase. Emerg Infect Dis 2001; 7(5): 910-1.
[http://dx.doi.org/10.3201/eid0705.010528] [PMID: 11747713]

[29]   Shokri D, Rabbani Khorasgani M, Zaghian S, *et al.* Determination of acquired resistance profiles of *Pseudomonas aeruginosa* isolates and characterization of an effective bacteriocin-like inhibitory substance (BLIS) against these isolates. Jundishapur J Microbiol 2016; 9(8): e32795.
[http://dx.doi.org/10.5812/jjm.32795] [PMID: 27800131]

[30]   Pang Z, Raudonis R, Glick BR, Lin T-J, Cheng Z. Antibiotic resistance in *Pseudomonas aeruginosa*: mechanisms and alternative therapeutic strategies. Biotechnol Adv 2019; 37(1): 177-92.
[http://dx.doi.org/10.1016/j.biotechadv.2018.11.013] [PMID: 30500353]

[31]   Walkty A, Adam H, Baxter M, *et al.* *In vitro* activity of plazomicin against 5,015 gram-negative and gram-positive clinical isolates obtained from patients in canadian hospitals as part of the CANWARD study, 2011-2012. Antimicrob Agents Chemother 2014; 58(5): 2554-63.
[http://dx.doi.org/10.1128/AAC.02744-13] [PMID: 24550325]

[32]   Aggen JB, Armstrong ES, Goldblum AA, *et al.* Synthesis and spectrum of the neoglycoside ACHN-490. Antimicrob Agents Chemother 2010; 54(11): 4636-42.
[http://dx.doi.org/10.1128/AAC.00572-10] [PMID: 20805391]

[33]   Reimann H, Cooper DJ, Mallams AK, *et al.* The structure of sisomicin, a novel unsaturated aminocyclitol antibiotic from Micromonospora inyoensis. J Org Chem 1974; 39(11): 1451-7.
[http://dx.doi.org/10.1021/jo00924a001] [PMID: 4833504]

[34]   Karaiskos I, Souli M, Giamarellou H. Plazomicin: an investigational therapy for the treatment of urinary tract infections. Expert Opin Investig Drugs 2015; 24(11): 1501-11.
[http://dx.doi.org/10.1517/13543784.2015.1095180] [PMID: 26419762]

[35]   Greer ND, Ed. Doripenem (Doribax): the newest addition to the carbapenems Baylor University Medical Center Proceedings. Taylor & Francis 2008.

[36]   Queenan AM, Shang W, Flamm R, Bush K. Hydrolysis and inhibition profiles of β-lactamases from molecular classes A to D with doripenem, imipenem, and meropenem. Antimicrob Agents Chemother 2010; 54(1): 565-9.
[http://dx.doi.org/10.1128/AAC.01004-09] [PMID: 19884379]

[37]   Cigana C, Bernardini F, Facchini M, *et al.* Efficacy of the novel antibiotic POL7001 in preclinical models of *Pseudomonas aeruginosa* pneumonia. Antimicrob Agents Chemother 2016; 60(8): 4991-5000.
[http://dx.doi.org/10.1128/AAC.00390-16] [PMID: 27297477]

[38]   Pappa O, Vantarakis A, Galanis A, Vantarakis G, Mavridou A. Antibiotic resistance profiles of *Pseudomonas aeruginosa* isolated from various Greek aquatic environments. FEMS Microbiol Ecol 2016; 92(6): fiw086.
[http://dx.doi.org/10.1093/femsec/fiw086] [PMID: 27146247]

[39]   Vidal F, Mensa J, Martínez JA, *et al.* *Pseudomonas aeruginosa* bacteremia in patients infected with human immunodeficiency virus type 1. Eur J Clin Microbiol Infect Dis 1999; 18(7): 473-7.
[http://dx.doi.org/10.1007/s100960050326] [PMID: 10482023]

[40]   Xu J, Duan X, Wu H, Zhou Q. Surveillance and correlation of antimicrobial usage and resistance of *Pseudomonas aeruginosa*: a hospital population-based study. PLoS One 2013; 8(11): e78604.
[http://dx.doi.org/10.1371/journal.pone.0078604] [PMID: 24250801]

[41]   Brooks G, Butel J, Morse S, Jawetz M. Adelberg's medical microbiology. Sultan Qaboos Univ Med J 2007; 7: 273.

[42]   Yadav R, Rogers KE, Bergen PJ, *et al.* Optimization and evaluation of piperacillin-tobramycin combination dosage regimens against *Pseudomonas aeruginosa* for patients with altered pharmacokinetics *via* the hollow-fiber infection model and mechanism-based modeling. Antimicrob Agents Chemother 2018; 62(5): e00078-18.
[http://dx.doi.org/10.1128/AAC.00078-18] [PMID: 29463528]

CHAPTER 8

Toxin-Antitoxin Systems

M. Mahmoudi[1], S. Ghafourian[1,*] and A. Maleki[2]

[1] *Department of Microbiology, Faculty of Medicine, Ilam University of Medical Sciences, Ilam, Iran*

[2] *Clinical Microbiology Research Center, Ilam University of Medical Sciences, Ilam, Iran*

Abstract: Toxin-antitoxin (TA) systems are found in large numbers in the bacterial genome. They were even seen as multiple copies in most cases. Structurally, TA systems are encoded by two or more adjacent genes that are expressed toxin and its cognate antitoxin elements all together. Generally, antitoxin neutralizes its cognate toxins and thus controls TA system functions. All toxins are protein elements while antitoxins can be proteins or non-coding RNAs. Hitherto, six types of TA systems are considered based on structural features and mode of action. Type II is more attractive to researchers due to its high frequency. Scientists believe that TA systems are involved in key biological functions due to their regulatory properties. Therefore, several crucial features have been proven for TA systems including, biofilm formation, persister cell formation, antibiotic resistance, programmed cell death, plasmid maintenance, *etc.* Since these systems are abundant, regulatory, and involved in the biology of bacteria, they have been studied as potent antimicrobial targets. The purpose of writing this chapter is to acquaint the reader with the different aspects of these systems to become more familiar with TA systems importance and performance.

Keywords: Antibiotic resistance, Biofilm, Persister cell, Plasmid maintenance, Post-segregational killing, Programmed cell death, Regulatory systems, Types of TA systems.

Teru Ogura and Sota Hiraga discovered the TA system in 1983. The discovery process happened when they observed a 700 bp segment of DNA that is very helpful for the propagation of mini-F plasmid compare to those with lack of mentioned DNA segment [1].

TA systems can be found in the genome of bacteria abundantly [2]. This issue made them attractive to many scientists. Because, due to occupying a significant volume of the genome by TA systems, they should play important roles in the

* **Corresponding author S. Ghafourian:** Department of Microbiology, Faculty of Medicine, Ilam University of Medical Sciences, Iran; E-mail: sobhan.ghafurian@gmail.com

Mina Mahmoudi, Sobhan Ghafourian & Behzad Badakhsh (Eds.)

biology of the bacteria. Based on this primary issue, several scientists focus on TA systems as we do.

Usually, TA systems consist of two genes that encode antitoxin and correspondingly toxin. In terms of structure, toxins are always made of protein. In contrast, the antitoxin can be made from protein or RNA. Most of the toxins have enzymatic activity and impress translation or DNA replication. In addition, antitoxin controls the activity of toxin [3].

In the normal mode (non-stress condition), antitoxin and toxin both are expressed in bacterial cell and antitoxin neutralizes toxin by forming TA complex [4]. In detail, antitoxin contrasts with toxin in several ways including, direct interaction, regulation of transcription or translation and cooperation with other signaling components [3].

Until now, several functions are allocated to TA system that some of them have great importance such as persister cell formation, post segregational killing (PSK) and abortive infection [4]. However, several other functions are considered for TA systems and we will explain them in the following.

Subsequently, TA system can be found in both chromosome and plasmid. The TA system, which located on plasmid causes a special phenotype named post segregation killing. During cell division, only daughter cells that inherit the plasmid will survive. In contrast, the daughter cell, which could not inherit the plasmid containing TA system, will be killed. The reason for this issue is associated with the instability of the antitoxin. Based on this, the stable toxin can kill the bacterial cell without any disturbance [5]. Another property of the TA system is plasmid stabilization. According to this property, being selfish is attributed to TA system. This feature is also related to PSK [6].

Chromosomal TA systems are less known due to the complexities of the chromosome. However, as it was mentioned, TA systems occupy a large part of the chromosome and large deletion of chromosomes is fatal for daughter cells.

Since antibiotic resistance is increasing dramatically, science has not been very successful in combating with microbial agents. Therefore, in recent years, scientists have been working hard to find new antibiotics and mostly new antimicrobial targets. One of the potent options is TA system, based on its regulatory properties.

On the other hand, the Infection Diseases Society of America (IDSA) introduced a group of most important and fatal bacterial pathogens, which are in urgent need of new treatments. This cohort of bacterial pathogens is named as ESKAPE, which demonstrates their ability to escape and defeat the treatment process. These pathogens are *Enterococcus faecium, S. aureus, K. pneumoniae, Acinetobacter baumannii, P. aeruginosa* and *Enterobacter* spp [7].

Therefore, TA systems become highly valuable according to the clinical importance of *P. aeruginosa* and potential microbial Targets of TA systems. Thus, understanding and studying TA systems is very important to overcome the problems caused by antibiotic resistance.

Given that, ParAB, TOX1/TOX2, T/AT1-2, HigBA, GraTA, MazEF, YefM/YoeB, Hha/TomB, PasTI, RelBE are some examples of TA systems that have been identified in *P. aeruginosa.* Also, TA systems are divided into different types, which we will explain later. However, all mentioned TA systems belong to type II and each of them has its own properties [8].

For more recognition, we will elucidate some functions of them briefly. ParAB, TOX1/TOX2, T/AT1-2 are located on the plasmid and they are involved in plasmid maintenance and carbapenem resistance [9]. HigBA can be found on both chromosome and plasmid Rts1. It is associated with the reduction of pyochelin, swarming and biofilm formation [10, 11]. GraTA, and MazEF are located on chromosome and they are involved in persister cell formation [12, 13]. Lastly, Hha/TomB, and yefM-yoeB are harbored by chromosome and correlated with the regulation of virulence [8].

1. CLASSIFICATION OF THE TA SYSTEMS

As of now, six types of TA systems are discovered (types I to VI). The principles of the classification are based on the manner of antitoxin to neutralize the toxin. In fact, there are four major TA systems. Among them, antitoxin of type I and type III are RNA molecules that can inhibit the toxin through two different manners. In details, it can regulate the level of active toxin (protein). In addition, it can inhibit the toxin protein of type III directly. However, in the other type of TA systems, the antitoxin and toxin are both proteins, which can interact with each other directly and easily. As well, the antitoxin is able to reverse the effect of the toxin on target molecules and compensate damages [14].

Besides, type V and type VI are recently discovered and are regarded as single modules [3].

1.1. Type I TA System

Type I TA system consists of antisense small RNA (sRNA) and stable mRNA toxin. Based on the main principle, the antitoxin neutralizes the toxin. But in detail, antitoxin sRNA pairs with the toxin mRNA and inhibits the expression of the toxin. It leads to inhibition of the base pairing between toxin mRNA and Shine-Dalgarno sequence. For more explanation, the ribosomal binding site in mRNA named Shine-Dalgarno sequence is located approximately 8 bases upstream of the start codon (AUG) and also plays an initial role in the synthesis of the protein *via* recruiting the ribosome to mRNA [14, 15]. Type I TA is highly toxic, so it quickly destroys the cell, which causes severe limitations to study about it. Therefore, the intracellular activity of the type I TA system is not well-known [16]. Structurally, type I toxin is shorter than 60 amino acids but is rich in hydrophobic proteins [17]. Type I TA system harbored on both plasmid and chromosome [18]. One of the most famous examples for type I is *hok/sok* TA system. Unusually, hok/sok locus also has a third component named mok. The *moke* gene overlaps with *hoke* gene, which contributes to the translation of toxin and kills the bacterial cell [19]. In addition, because of this overlapping, the antitoxin can also pair with the third component and prevent the translation of the toxin [20].

In addition, ldr/Rdl, tisB/IstR1, ibs/Sib, shoB/OhsC and symE/SymR are some examples of the type I TA system [16].

1.2. Type II TA System

Type II is the most prevalent TA system among bacteria. Also, the antitoxin and toxin are both proteins. The type II operon consists of two genes with approximately 80-630 bp long. Also, there is a small fragment that can separate these two genes. Sometimes, this small fragment causes overlaps of antitoxin and toxin genes. In addition, this small fragment can be located from –20 to +30 nucleotides [21]. In normal conditions, the antitoxin and toxin form TA complex and toxin will be neutralized. But, as the antitoxin is unstable, environmental changes can arouse its' regulatory properties. Therefore, the antitoxin will be destroyed by the activation of Lon and Clp proteases. As a result, the transcription of the operon will be started which leads to the production of a high level of free toxin and kills the bacterial cell [22].

In particular, the most popular activity of toxin type II is endonuclease or interferase activity [23]. In addition, some well-known intracellular targets of the toxin type II are DNA gyrase, ribosome, elongation factor thermal unstable or uridine diphosphate-N-acetylglucosamine [24].

More classifications can be found in the type II TA system. To date, there are three main groups of type II TA systems that are confirmed in *S. aureus* including, MazEF/PemIK, YefM-YoeB (AxeTxe) and Omega-Epsilon-Zeta.

MazEF was firstly found in the chromosome of *E. coli* and is located in *rsbUVWsigB* locus. MazEF TA system causes bacterial sacrifice through induction of programmed cell death (PCD). For more clarity, by starvation of amino acids, the protease enzymes degrade the antitoxin, which leads to the accumulation of free toxin. When the toxin killed the bacteria, its constituents are released into the environment and other bacteria will uptake them. In this way, some bacteria kill themselves *via* mazEF TA system, which assists other bacteria to survive and the bacterial population to be maintained [25].

On the other hand, pemIKsa system was discovered on the plasmid pCH91. It is highly similar to mazEF but some of its amino acids are different. It can be found on both plasmid and chromosome of some staphylococcal species. The toxin PemKsa has RNase activity and interferes with cell growth. The antitoxin PemI can neutralize the toxin PemKsa [26].

The second group is YefM-YoeB TA system. YoeB is a toxin and YefM is an antitoxin that is evolutionarily associated with RelE and Phd, respectively [27]. The target of YoeB is the ribosome and causes cleavage of the mRNA [28]. The Axe-Txe is regarded as the homolog of the YefM-YoeB that can be found in the plasmid of *Enterococcus* spp [29].

The third group consists of three components, Omega/Epsilon/Zeta. Epsilon is an antitoxin that can inhibit the activity of toxin Zeta and Omega that can regulate the operon. Zeta toxin causes autolysis. In detail, uridine diphosphate-N-acetylglucosamine is a peptidoglycan precursor, which Zeta toxin can phosphorylate it and this leads to the prevention of peptidoglycan synthesis. So, the bacteria will be autolyzed [7].

1.3. Type III TA System

Here, the antitoxin is RNA and the toxin is a protein similar to the type I TA system. The bioinformatics analysis identified more than 100 type II TA systems among bacteria [30]. toxI/toxN is described as the first Type III TA system that was located on plasmid pECA1039. The ability of *Pectobacterium carotovoum* to be resistant against bacteriophage infection was related to toxI/toxN and conducted the discovery of Type III TA system [31]. Although, type I and III TA system are similar in terms of the material of components, they are different in the mode of interaction. So, antitoxin directly neutralizes toxin by binding in the type I TA system [32].

But, in type III the neutralization process is more complicated. More precisely, *toxN* gene preceded by other parts, a short inverted repeat that is preceded by a tandem array of direct repeats. The short inverted repeat act as the transcriptional terminator. It controls the amount of antitoxic sRNA and toxin mRNA transcription. The toxin is ToxN and the antitoxin is ToxI.

The direct repeat is a target of RNase activity of ToxN and it will cleave the transcript of toxI/toxN. As a result, the RNA antitoxin will be free having 36 nt length [19, 33].

Subsequently, the interaction between antitoxin sRNA and toxin protein forms ToxIN complex. This complex has a very intricate structure. Hence, in an overview, it has a heterohexameric triangular structure. So, it is composed of three ToxN proteins, which are separated by three 36 nt ToxI sRNA pseudo-knots [34].

1.4. Type IV TA System

Unlike other systems, the antitoxin and toxin of the type IV TA system are not binding with each other directly. Also, they are not abundant. One of the most famous TA systems in this type is YeeUV (Later, the name changed to cbeA/cbtA)and can be found in *E. coli*. As was mentioned, the antitoxin and toxin of this type are not binding to each other directly, but the antitoxin stabilizes the cellular targets of the toxin [35]. So, for better understanding, we first introduce cellular targets of the toxin. FtsZ and MreB prokaryotic proteins are both in the structure of the cytoskeleton. The FtsZ protein is the homolog of tubulin that contributes to cell division.

This is the first protein that locates at the site of the cell division and forms the Z ring. The formation of Z ring leads to the activation of more than ten proteins that are involved in the development of cytokinesis [36]. On the other hand, the MreB is an actin-like protein and is necessary to preserve the rod shape of the bacterial cell. It has other functions including, cell division, and dissociation of the chromosome and cell polarity [37].

Therefore, the YeeV (CbtA) toxin affects FtsZ and MreB proteins and prevents cell growth. For these reasons, a group of scientists proposed CbeA instead of YeeU due to the bundling-enhancing factor A activity [38]. Based on this for the neutralization purpose, the CbeA is an antitoxin that neutralizes the effects of toxin CbtA by stabilization of MreB and FtsZ [21].

1.5. Type V TA System

The type V TA system is discovered recently and it is unique compared with previous TA systems. GhoS/GhoT TA system is categorized in the type V TA system. GhoS is an antitoxin and GhoT is a toxin [21]. GhoS has a particular sequence that has endoribonuclease activity against mRNA of GhoT toxin. So, the target of GhoS is mRNA of toxin and inhibits the translation of toxin. However, toxin protein expression occurs interestingly [39]. The GhoS/GhoT TA system is not independent. Another TA system, MqsRA, also controls the level of the mRNA of GhoS. Therefore, by the degradation of GhoS (antitoxin) mRNA through MqsR, the mRNA of GhoT(toxin) can survive and produce toxin protein [40].

1.6. Type VI TA System

This is a novel TA system that both antitoxin and toxin are composed of protein. One of the obvious examples of this type is SocAB system. SocA and SocB are antitoxin and toxin, respectively. The effect of antitoxin is indirectly as same as type IV TA system, but with a different mechanism. In fact, SocA is an adaptor of ClpXP protease that can degrade SocB. This process was found in *Caulobacter crescentus* [41]. In addition, at the time of toxin activity, replication of cells will be blocked *via* binding to β sliding clamp DnaN [42]. For more clarity, the sliding clamp factor is located in the structure of DNA polymerase III and boosts DNA replication. In fact, the clamping factor prevents from separation of DNA polymerase III and DNA template. Thus, by attaching toxin to the sliding clamp, the DNA polymerase III is not able to continue the replication [43].

2. TA SYSTEM FUNCTIONS

Since TA systems play an important role in the pathogenicity of bacteria, we will explain their role in the pathogenesis and regulation of bacterial genes in the following.

2.1. Antibiotic Resistance

One of the most important and detailed effects of the TA systems on the bacterial population is the development and maintenance of antibiotic resistance [44, 45]. As it is obvious, there are several roles of TA systems involved in antibiotic resistance including, plasmid maintenance, biofilm formation, persister cell formation, *etc* [46]. Here, we will give you a comprehensive explanation of the association between the mentioned roles of TA systems and antibiotic resistance. Nevertheless, each of these roles is also explained as a separate part of the following.

The transformation of the conjugate plasmid can cause antibiotic resistance by the transfer of resistance genes. This feature can significantly increase bacterial survival and cause serious health problems for humans [47]. However, bacterial success in survival is not only limited to obtaining resistance genes. Since plasmids are extra-chromosomal genetic elements, they cause a metabolic burden on bacterial cells [48]. Therefore, bacterial cells will maintain the plasmid as long as they expose to the antibiotic. But when the antibiotic is removed from the environment, the bacterial cell does not need a plasmid containing the resistance gene to survive. Therefore, it loses the plasmid to reduce metabolic burden. As a result, bacterial cells only maintain plasmids until they need them otherwise, they will be eliminated. Accordingly, if the bacterial cell encounters the same antibiotic again, it will die [49]. Although bacteria protect themselves in this way but it does not guarantee long-term survival. TA systems are one of the most effective ways to maintain the plasmid in the bacterial population permanently through selective internal pressure. This process is one of the most important functions of TA systems called plasmid maintenance [50]. Here, we briefly explain the mechanism of plasmid maintenance by TA systems but the details are available in the following (8.2.7 Plasmid maintenance). As mentioned earlier, TA systems consist of stable toxin and its cognate labile antitoxin that can inhibit the toxin [51]. Supposing that there is bacterial cell, which contains a plasmid that has TA system and antibiotic resistance genes both together. The toxin and labile antitoxin are expressed simultaneously and toxin inhibited by the antitoxin. At the time of the cell division, one of the daughter cells obtains the plasmid and but not the other one. The daughter cell, which obtains the plasmid, the toxin and antitoxin expresses together. But, the other daughter cell that the plasmid was not inherited only obtain toxin and antitoxin molecules in the cytoplasm of the bacterial cell. The antitoxin is labile, so, after a short time, only the stable toxin remains and kills the bacterial cell. By this way, TA system maintains the plasmid, which harbored the antibiotic resistance genes even in the absence of the antibiotic in the environment. In conclusion, during bacterial growth, only cells that contain the plasmid (carrying an antibiotic resistance gene) remain in the bacterial population through TA system function [49]. Thus, TA systems influence antibiotic resistance. For instance, Hok/sok and CcdAB systems are responsible for plasmid maintenance, which can also be influenced in antibiotic resistance [52, 53].

TA systems also influence biofilm formation. In order to better understanding, initially, we will explain how biofilm causes antibiotic resistance and then, how the TA system regulates biofilm formation.

The biofilm is a complex structure that enclosed bacterial cells and acts as a barrier against environmental factors [54]. Therefore, antibiotics face a great challenge to reach their targets. Many antibiotics fail to enter into the biofilm structure at the beginning. However, in the high concentration of the antibiotics, some of them enter into the biofilm. However, inside the biofilm structure, there are other mechanisms of antibiotic resistance. *P. aeruginosa* produces the strongest biofilm among bacterial and low levels of the β-lactamase. Since biofilm is a closed structure, the concentration of β-lactamase slowly increases inside of biofilm and it will be more effective against β-lactam antibiotics [55]. On the other hand, some constituent molecules of biofilm have negative charge including, alginate and eDNA [56]. In contrast, some of the antibiotics have a positive charge such as aminoglycosides [57]. Alginate and eDNA sequester the aminoglycosides and prevent them from deep penetration into the biofilm [58, 59]. In addition, biofilm provides anaerobic conditions, which reduces the effect of aminoglycosides. However, the level of biofilm resistance depends on the type of antibiotic [60]. Eventually, based on what has been described, biofilm causes antibiotic resistance [61].

As of now, many TA systems present as regulon of biofilm including, MgsRA, MazEF, RelBE [62 - 64]. The regulation of the biofilm through TA systems is fully explained in the following (8.2.2 Biofilm formation). However, here, it will be explained briefly in order to better understanding of antibiotic resistance through biofilm.

Some genes are involved in the biofilm, which regulates *via* quorum sensing [65]. QseBC is a two-component (B and C) regulatory system in *E. coli*, which regulates motility and flagella that leads to the biofilm dispersion [66, 67]. For this purpose, QseBC controls another master regulator; *flhDC,* that regulates the movement of the flagellum [68]. *mqsR*, the toxin of MqsRA TA system, regulates *qseBC* and subsequently *flhDC*, which leads to the induction of biofilm [69].In addition, Autoinducer-2 (AI-2), a signal molecule *in E. coli*, regulates the biofilm and motility through *mqsR* and *motA,* respectively [70]. *motA* encodes motility protein MotA that is located in the flagellum structure [71]. Taken together, one of the reasons for antibiotic resistance is biofilm formation that could be regulated *via* TA system.

Moreover, another cause of bacterial resistance is persister cell formation, which is also can be found in biofilm. Persister cells account for about 1% of some bacterial populations that highly persist to antibacterial agents. Persister cells form spontaneously and are metabolically inactive [72]. *P. aeruginosa* is able to form persister cells, which is documented in cystic fibrosis patients [73]. TA systems are also able to regulate persister cell formation by dormancy induction. This statement makes cells persistent in the effect of antibiotics and antibacterial agents [74]. Indeed, environmental stress induces persister cell formation such as DNA damage, lack or shortage of nutrients and extreme pH. It seems that the reason for persister cell formation in the depth of biofilm is a nutrient limitation [75]. Many

TA systems also influence the regulation of persister cells including, mazEF, RelBE, HipBA, *etc* [13, 76]. However, the association of TA systems and persister cell formation is completely explained in the following (8.2.3 Persister cell formation).

2.2. Biofilm Formation

As it was mentioned, biofilm formation is highly associated with chronic infection and antibiotic resistance. Hence, by the resistance of bacteria to the immune host defense, it can convert to a dangerous human pathogen like *P. aeruginosa* and *Mycobacterium tuberculosis* [77]. In addition, the biofilm is also regarded as the host of persister cells [78].

One of the most important TA systems that have a direct role in biofilm formation is MqSRA. Also, MqsR is toxin andMqsA is antitoxin in this module.

In 2006, Gonzalez Barrios *et al.* studied the role of MqsR in biofilm formation in *E. coli*. The MqsR encoded by b3022 that causes eight folds in biofilm. Also, b3022 gene changed its name to *MqsR*.It has been proven that MqsR controls the biofilm formation in *E. coli*, but the mechanism needs some more explanation. Hence, there is flagella and motility regulator in the chromosome of *E. coli*, QseBC, which is associated with quorum sensing. QseB is a response regulator and QseCis the sensor kinase. There is another master regulator flhDC, which is under the control of the QseBC. FlhDC regulates the movement of the flagellum by three specific genes, *fliC, fliA,* and *motA*. More precisely, *fliC* encodes the major flagellin protein, *fliA* encodes sigma factor and *motA* causes flagellum movement [70]. Indeed, the regulation of motility has a very crucial role in the formation of the biofilm. Since in the initial stage of the biofilm formation, the flagella motility provides swimming motility and assists to reach the desired surface. Then, the planktonic bacteria should convert to a sessile biofilm state. All of these events are under the control of the quorum sensing by changing the regulation of the motility [79]. Based on this, the MqsR controls biofilm formation by induction of QseBC through positive regulation.

On the other hand, the autoinducer 2 controls biofilm formation in *E. coli via* MqsR and also stimulates motility of the bacteria through *motA*. In other words, MqsRA acts as a mediator for AI-2 and motility [70].

As it was mentioned, MqsrA is antitoxin of this system and it is also involved in biofilm formation but with another mechanism. MqsrA represses the expression of RpoS and CsgD, which are stress response regulators. As a result, signaling of the nucleotide c-di-GMP will decrease; as well,the production of curli also comes down. Finally, biofilm formation will reduce [80].

But, in the oxidative stress condition, the Lon protease degrades MqsA that leads to the increasing of biofilm formation [81].

On the other hand, the mazEF TA system is also involved in biofilm survival. As it was mentioned the mazEF causes PCD, so when the bacteria face amino acid deficiency, the mazEF kills a part of the bacterial population. In this way, the structural components of the killed bacteria will be available to other bacterial populations. As a result, the bacterial population of the biofilm will be survived [82].

2.3. Persister Cell Formation

Persister cells are a small population of bacteria that are dormant and forms stochastically. The remarkable point about the persister cells is their ability to tolerate plenty amount of antibiotics [83]. In a simple word, they are immortal bacterial cells that are formed for no apparent reason. As of now, many TA systems have been identified that their toxins are highly induced in persister cells such as mqsR, relE, higB, mazF, yafQ, and yoeB [76, 84, 85].

For better understanding, we will explain the role of TisAB/IstR-1 TA system in the formation of the persister cells of *E. coli* in the following. One of the popular antibiotics for the treatment of infections caused by *E. coli* is ciprofloxacin [86]. Ciprofloxacin targets are DNA gyrase, type II and V topoisomerase. It also contributes to the separation of bacterial DNA that leads to preventing cell division [87]. As a point, any kind of DNA damage triggers SOS response system, which repairs the DNA. The lexA protein is a repressor of the SOS response and the RecA is an inducer, which is sensitive to single-stranded DNA (ssDNA) and activates the system through lexA cleavage [88].

TisAB/IstR-1 TA influenced in persister cell by induction of tisB toxin. TisAB/IstR-1 contains IstR-1, IstR-2 (sRNA) and TisAB, a toxic part that is under the control of lexA. Therefore, TisAB can be activated by SOS response. Also, SOS response regulates the transcription of IstR-2. IstR-1 is an antitoxin that can neutralize the TisB by biding to the LexA and induction of the RNAase III [89]. Here, the RNAse III prevents the expression of TisB by cleavage of TisB mRNA.

In the normal mode (no DNA damage), istR-1 is produced abundantly and induces RNAase III, which leads to the cleavage of tisB mRNA and eliminates the toxicity caused by TisAB [90].

As it was mentioned, ciprofloxacin copes with the bacteria by DNA damage that leads to the activation of SOS response. In a simple word, high amounts of ssDNA activate the RecA that leads to the cleavage of lexA and SOS response will be triggered. Here, the antitoxin IstR-1 cannot bind to lexA to inhibit the TisB expression, because, by the activation of SOS response, lexA is completely cleaved. Therefore, the level of TisB will be increased. Subsequently, TisB binds to the cytoplasmic membrane. This binding leads to membrane damage and decreasing the level of protein motive force and ATP [91]. Given that, the level of the materials that are essential for cell growth including DNA, RNA, and protein comes down. Therefore, bacteria are not able to absorb antibiotics as normal mode, as well;the cell goes to the dormant phase. Eventually, by this mechanism, the persister cells will emerge Fig. (**1**) [92].

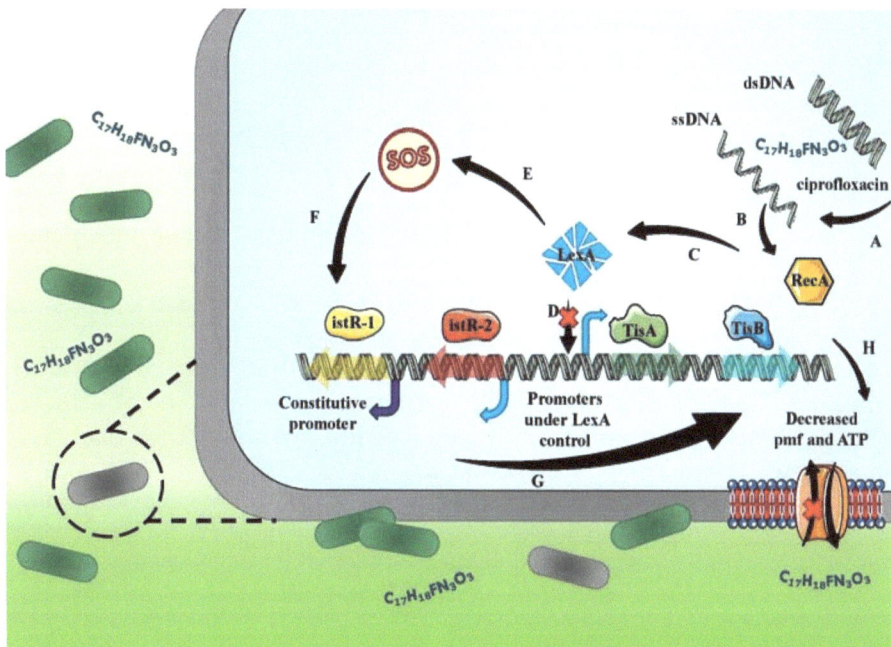

Fig. (1). Persister cell formation. (**A**) Ciprofloxacin, a fluoroquinolone, is one of the antibiotics that affect bacterial DNA and kills the bacterium by converting dsDNA to ssDNA. (**B**) on the other hand, RecA protein, which belongs to the SOS response system, the general response to DNA damages, stimulated by the accumulation of ssDNA inside the cell. (**C**) the RecA protein interacted with the LexA, the repressor of SOS response, which leads to the cleavage of LexA. (**D**) promoters under the control of the LexA will be uncontrolled. (**E**) on the other hand, by the degradation of the LexA, the SOS response genes will be activated, which triggers the DNA repair process. (**F**) Besides, induction of the SOS response leads to the cleavage of istR-1, which controlled the amount of the toxin TisB. (**G**) by the degradation of the IstR-1, the expression of the tisB will be started. (**H**) finally, TisB binds to the cytoplasmic membrane that leads to the membrane damage and depression of pmf and ATP. So, bacterial cell doesn't able to absorb antibiotics, which leads cell to dormant or persister form.

2.4. Genomic Junk

Junk function is a gene non-coding transfer from plasmid or other sources to chromosome, which are regulated by TA loci [92].

2.5. Programmed Cell Death (PCD)

One of the most known TA systems for PCD is MazEF that is belonging to type II. There are four genes within relA operon in *E. coli* MC4100 including, *relA*, *mazE*, *mazF* and, *mazG*. In addition, there are three promoters in relA operon, P1, P2 and, P3. When the transcription occurs from P2 and p3 promoter, MazEF mRNA will be produced. Then, it will be translating, which leads to the formation of MazEF complex. MazEF complex contains four MazE *versus* two MazF (+ +). The complex of MazEF followed two pathways. On one hand, it can directly repress the activation of the mentioned genes. On the other hand, clpAP serine protease cleaves the antitoxin MazE that leads to the liberation of the toxin MazF. The intracellular target of the toxin is cellular RNA that will be cleaved by the toxic property of MazF.

Finally, the cell goes to death [82], but how MazE is degraded by clpAP serine protease?

The answer to this question is related to the sacrifice characterization among bacteria that can happen *via* TA systems. In the time of amino acid starvation, clpAP serine protease will be activated and traps the antitoxin MazE. So, toxin MazF assails to the cells freely and kills them. By this process, other bacteria within the population can obtain nutrients that are released from the carcass of other bacteria. Although, some of the bacteria will be killed in this way but the rest of the population survive and the bacterial population will be saved [93].

2.6. Post Segregational killing (PSK)

This function is related to the TA systems that are harbored in the plasmid. Obviously, the toxin is a stable protein while the antitoxin is an unstable component. They are both expressed inside the bacterial cell and the antitoxin neutralizes the toxin. When the TA system locates in the plasmid, only the daughter cell that obtains that plasmid inherits TA systems properties. For more clarity, one of the daughter cells inherits plasmid (TA system) toxin and antitoxin. The other one inherits only toxin and antitoxin. As the antitoxin is unstable, it will be degraded. So, this daughter cell goes to death *via* activation of the free toxin. In contrast, the other daughter cell that obtains the plasmid will be survived. But why? Because toxin and antitoxin are both expressed and the antitoxin neutralized the toxin due to the presence of TA system in the mentioned plasmid (Fig. **2**) [94, 95].

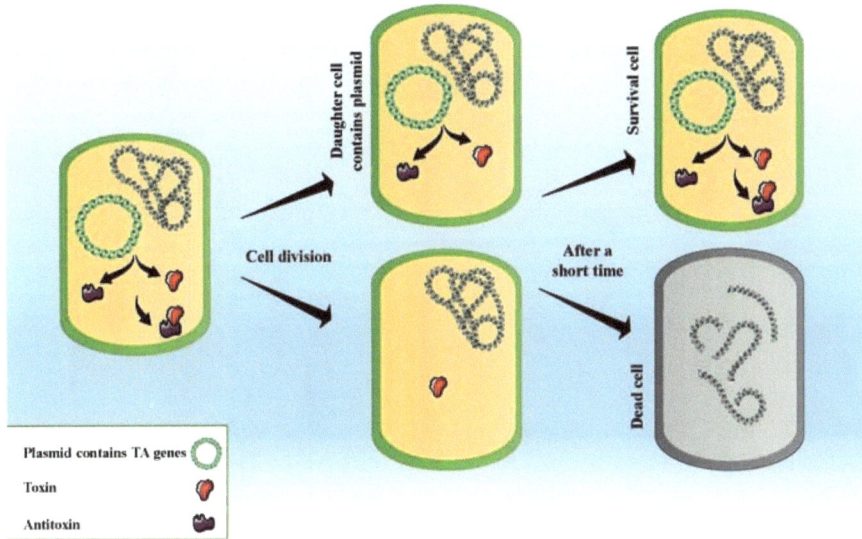

Fig. (2). Post Segregational killing (PSK). **(A)**: Mother cell contains TA system: PSK function is related to the TA systems, which are located on plasmids. Toxin and antitoxin expressed from the plasmid and antitoxin neutralized the toxin effect. So, the mother cell continued to its life and reproduced. **(B)**: After the cell division, only one of the daughter cells inherits the plasmid but both of them inherit Intracellular materials that included toxins and antitoxins. As the antitoxin is unstable, it will be degraded. In contrast, Toxin is stable and without the presence of antitoxin, it becomes a threat to the bacterial cell. The daughter cell that inherits the plasmid acts like the mother cell, and the system is neutralized by the simultaneous expression of antitoxins and toxins. **(C)**: After a short time in a cell without plasmid, the toxin reaches its target and exerts a deadly effect. Therefore, the cell without plasmid is destroyed. As a result, the plasmid containing the TA system is preserved in the bacterial population.

2.7. Plasmid Maintenance

The plasmid maintenance is associated with vertical gene transfer. By the absence of the plasmid that harbored the TA system in the daughter cell, unstable antitoxin will be degraded and the toxin kills the cell. In contrast, only the daughter cell that obtains the plasmid will be alive due to the production of the toxin and antitoxin. Accordingly, the presence of TA system gene in plasmid inhibits the destruction of the cell. So, by the presence of the plasmid, the daughter cell will be alive, as well plasmid will be maintained [49].

2.8. Antiphage Activity

Although bacteria are one of the most important infectious agents, they are also susceptible to infection. Therefore, the bacteriophage is one of the bacterial pathogens that can be highly effective against bacteria [96]. In order to deal with this problem, several defense systems are embedded in bacteria that cause resistance against bacteriophage. Here are some examples of these defense mechanisms, preventing absorption at the bacterial surface, super infection exclusion, cleavage of phage nucleic acid (CRISPR-Cas system) and abortive infection [97 - 100].

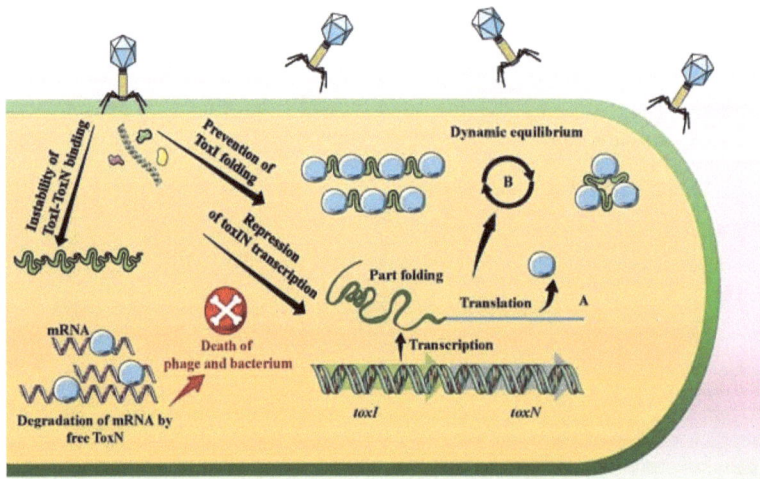

Fig. (3). Antiphage activity. **(A)** In the normal mode, *toxIN* transcribed constitutively and then, *toxI* single repeats folded and forms RNA pseudoknots. Besides, ToxN proteins formed by translation. **(B)** ToxN changed the full-length ToxI RNA structure and formed a stable trimeric complex with it. On the other hand, new full-length ToxI RNA can deflect ToxN of a trimeric complex, which causes a dynamic balance between them. Under high expression conditions, this balance moved to the right due to the presents of a high amount of full-length ToxI RNA **(C)** with the onset of viral infection, this pathway is impaired through viral components. In general, a viral infection caused repression of the *toxIN* transcription, prevention of ToxI folding, and instability of ToxI-ToxN binding, which leads to the ToxN liberation. As it was mentioned, the trimeric toxIN complex is not the dominant form under the high expression condition. Therefore, the activation of ToxN is not probably due to the separation of ToxN from the trimeric complex. **(D)** the intracellular target of ToxN is mRNA. So, if a significant amount of ToxN is released into the cell, the host bacterial cell and the phage will be destroyed. This cell defense mechanism is called abortive infection.

Bacterial abortive infection system is described as altruistic behavior, which results in bacterial death. Therefore, by the suicide of infected bacteria, the phage loses its host. Thus, the phage replication cycle will be disrupted and limited.

Also, premature phages die and they are not able to spread anymore. So, the bacterial population will be survived. Hitherto, several TA systems are known that they have antiphage activity including, Hok-Sok (type I), LosAB and MazEF (type II), ToxIN (type III) and AbiEG (type IV). Here we will describe how ToxIN deals with incoming phage.

In the normal mode, antitoxin and toxin genes are both transcribed. Then, antitoxin ToxI forms RNA pseudoknots. Then, ToxI and ToxN form a terimeric TA complex. But, there is a dynamic balance between ToxI and ToxN that causes formation, slightly.

By the way, in the presence of phage components, this pathway is impaired. So, the transcription of the ToxIN will be suppressed and also the antitoxins that are present inside the bacterial cell cannot be properly folded. In addition, the binding of antitoxin and toxin also becomes unstable. Eventually, the free toxin ToxN attacks its cellular targets. Here, the intracellular target of the ToxN is mRNA. So, by the destruction of the mRNAs, phage and host both go to death and this is how the abortive infection is formed (Fig. **3**) [101].

CONSENT FOR PUBLICATION

Not applicable.

CONFLICT OF INTEREST

The authors declare no conflict of interest, financial or otherwise.

ACKNOWLEDGEMENTS

Declared none.

REFERENCES

[1]   Ogura T, Hiraga S. Mini-F plasmid genes that couple host cell division to plasmid proliferation. Proc Natl Acad Sci USA 1983; 80(15): 4784-8.
        [http://dx.doi.org/10.1073/pnas.80.15.4784] [PMID: 6308648]

[2]   Saavedra De Bast M, Mine N, Van Melderen L. Chromosomal toxin-antitoxin systems may act as antiaddiction modules. J Bacteriol 2008; 190(13): 4603-9.
        [http://dx.doi.org/10.1128/JB.00357-08] [PMID: 18441063]

[3]   Harms A, Brodersen DE, Mitarai N, Gerdes K. Toxins, targets, and triggers: an overview of toxin-antitoxin biology. Mol Cell 2018; 70(5): 768-84.
        [http://dx.doi.org/10.1016/j.molcel.2018.01.003] [PMID: 29398446]

[4]   Rocker A, Meinhart A. Type II toxin: antitoxin systems. More than small selfish entities? Curr Genet 2016; 62(2): 287-90.
        [http://dx.doi.org/10.1007/s00294-015-0541-7] [PMID: 26597447]

[5]   Ogura T, Hiraga S. Partition mechanism of F plasmid: two plasmid gene-encoded products and a cis-

acting region are involved in partition. Cell 1983; 32(2): 351-60.
[http://dx.doi.org/10.1016/0092-8674(83)90454-3] [PMID: 6297791]

[6]   Cooper TF, Heinemann JA. Postsegregational killing does not increase plasmid stability but acts to mediate the exclusion of competing plasmids. Proc Natl Acad Sci USA 2000; 97(23): 12643-8.
[http://dx.doi.org/10.1073/pnas.220077897] [PMID: 11058151]

[7]   Aizenman E, Engelberg-Kulka H, Glaser G. An *Escherichia coli* chromosomal "addiction module" regulated by guanosine [corrected] 3′,5′-bispyrophosphate: a model for programmed bacterial cell death. Proc Natl Acad Sci USA 1996; 93(12): 6059-63.
[http://dx.doi.org/10.1073/pnas.93.12.6059] [PMID: 8650219]

[8]   Fernández-García L, Blasco L, Lopez M, *et al.* Toxin-antitoxin systems in clinical pathogens. Toxins (Basel) 2016; 8(7): 227.
[http://dx.doi.org/10.3390/toxins8070227] [PMID: 27447671]

[9]   Bonnin RA, Poirel L, Nordmann P, *et al.* Complete sequence of broad-host-range plasmid pNOR-2000 harbouring the metallo-β-lactamase gene blaVIM-2 from *Pseudomonas aeruginosa*. J Antimicrob Chemother 2013; 68(5): 1060-5.
[http://dx.doi.org/10.1093/jac/dks526] [PMID: 23354281]

[10]   Williams JJ, Halvorsen EM, Dwyer EM, DiFazio RM, Hergenrother PJ. Toxin-antitoxin (TA) systems are prevalent and transcribed in clinical isolates of *Pseudomonas aeruginosa* and methicillin-resistant *Staphylococcus aureus*. FEMS Microbiol Lett 2011; 322(1): 41-50.
[http://dx.doi.org/10.1111/j.1574-6968.2011.02330.x] [PMID: 21658105]

[11]   Wood TL, Wood TK. The HigB/HigA toxin/antitoxin system of *Pseudomonas aeruginosa* influences the virulence factors pyochelin, pyocyanin, and biofilm formation. MicrobiologyOpen 2016; 5(3): 499-511.
[http://dx.doi.org/10.1002/mbo3.346] [PMID: 26987441]

[12]   Ainelo A, Tamman H, Leppik M, Remme J, Hõrak R. The toxin GraT inhibits ribosome biogenesis. Mol Microbiol 2016; 100(4): 719-34.
[http://dx.doi.org/10.1111/mmi.13344] [PMID: 26833678]

[13]   Cho J, Carr AN, Whitworth L, Johnson B, Wilson KS. MazEF toxin-antitoxin proteins alter *Escherichia coli* cell morphology and infrastructure during persister formation and regrowth. Microbiology (Reading) 2017; 163(3): 308-21.
[http://dx.doi.org/10.1099/mic.0.000436] [PMID: 28113053]

[14]   Van Melderen L, Saavedra De Bast M. Bacterial toxin-antitoxin systems: more than selfish entities? PLoS Genet 2009; 5(3): e1000437.
[http://dx.doi.org/10.1371/journal.pgen.1000437] [PMID: 19325885]

[15]   Starmer J, Stomp A, Vouk M, Bitzer D. Predicting Shine-Dalgarno sequence locations exposes genome annotation errors. PLOS Comput Biol 2006; 2(5): e57.
[http://dx.doi.org/10.1371/journal.pcbi.0020057] [PMID: 16710451]

[16]   Wagner EGH, Unoson C. The toxin-antitoxin system tisB-istR1: Expression, regulation, and biological role in persister phenotypes. RNA Biol 2012; 9(12): 1513-9.
[http://dx.doi.org/10.4161/rna.22578] [PMID: 23093802]

[17]   Fozo EM, Makarova KS, Shabalina SA, Yutin N, Koonin EV, Storz G. Abundance of type I toxin-antitoxin systems in bacteria: searches for new candidates and discovery of novel families. Nucleic Acids Res 2010; 38(11): 3743-59.
[http://dx.doi.org/10.1093/nar/gkq054] [PMID: 20156992]

[18]   Fozo EM. New type I toxin-antitoxin families from "wild" and laboratory strains of *E. coli*: Ibs-Sib, ShoB-OhsC and Zor-Orz. RNA Biol 2012; 9(12): 1504-12.
[http://dx.doi.org/10.4161/rna.22568] [PMID: 23182878]

[19]   Ghafourian S, Raftari M, Sadeghifard N, Sekawi Z. Toxin-antitoxin systems: classification, biological

function and application in biotechnology. Curr Issues Mol Biol 2014; 16(1): 9-14.
[PMID: 23652423]

[20]   Gerdes K. Hypothesis: type I toxin–antitoxin genes enter the persistence field—a feedback mechanism explaining membrane homoeostasis. Philosophical Transactions of the Royal Society B: Biological Sciences 2016; 371(1707): 20160189.

[21]   Klimina K, Poluektova E, Danilenko V. Bacterial toxin–antitoxin systems: Properties, functional significance, and possibility of use. Appl Biochem Microbiol 2017; 53(5): 494-505.
[http://dx.doi.org/10.1134/S0003683817050076]

[22]   Muthuramalingam M, White JC, Bourne CR. Toxin-antitoxin modules are pliable switches activated by multiple protease pathways. Toxins (Basel) 2016; 8(7): 214.
[http://dx.doi.org/10.3390/toxins8070214] [PMID: 27409636]

[23]   Christensen-Dalsgaard M, Overgaard M, Winther KS, Gerdes K. RNA decay by messenger RNA interferases. Methods Enzymol 2008; 447: 521-35.
[http://dx.doi.org/10.1016/S0076-6879(08)02225-8] [PMID: 19161859]

[24]   Butt A, Müller C, Harmer N, Titball RW. Identification of type II toxin-antitoxin modules in Burkholderia pseudomallei. FEMS Microbiol Lett 2013; 338(1): 86-94.
[http://dx.doi.org/10.1111/1574-6968.12032] [PMID: 23082999]

[25]   Schuster CF, Bertram R. Toxin-antitoxin systems of *Staphylococcus aureus*. Toxins (Basel) 2016; 8(5): 140.
[http://dx.doi.org/10.3390/toxins8050140] [PMID: 27164142]

[26]   Bukowski M, Lyzen R, Helbin WM, *et al.* A regulatory role for *Staphylococcus aureus* toxin-antitoxin system PemIKSa. Nat Commun 2013; 4(1): 2012.
[http://dx.doi.org/10.1038/ncomms3012] [PMID: 23774061]

[27]   Hayes F, Kędzierska B. Regulating toxin-antitoxin expression: controlled detonation of intracellular molecular timebombs. Toxins (Basel) 2014; 6(1): 337-58.
[http://dx.doi.org/10.3390/toxins6010337] [PMID: 24434949]

[28]   Feng S, Chen Y, Kamada K, *et al.* YoeB-ribosome structure: a canonical RNase that requires the ribosome for its specific activity. Nucleic Acids Res 2013; 41(20): 9549-56.
[http://dx.doi.org/10.1093/nar/gkt742] [PMID: 23945936]

[29]   Grady R, Hayes F. Axe-Txe, a broad-spectrum proteic toxin-antitoxin system specified by a multidrug-resistant, clinical isolate of Enterococcus faecium. Mol Microbiol 2003; 47(5): 1419-32.
[http://dx.doi.org/10.1046/j.1365-2958.2003.03387.x] [PMID: 12603745]

[30]   Blower TR, Short FL, Rao F, *et al.* Identification and classification of bacterial Type III toxin-antitoxin systems encoded in chromosomal and plasmid genomes. Nucleic Acids Res 2012; 40(13): 6158-73.
[http://dx.doi.org/10.1093/nar/gks231] [PMID: 22434880]

[31]   Fineran PC, Blower TR, Foulds IJ, Humphreys DP, Lilley KS, Salmond GP. The phage abortive infection system, ToxIN, functions as a protein-RNA toxin-antitoxin pair. Proc Natl Acad Sci USA 2009; 106(3): 894-9.
[http://dx.doi.org/10.1073/pnas.0808832106] [PMID: 19124776]

[32]   Brantl S. Bacterial type I toxin-antitoxin systems. Taylor & Francis 2012.
[http://dx.doi.org/10.4161/rna.23045]

[33]   Unterholzner SJ, Poppenberger B, Rozhon W. Toxin-antitoxin systems: Biology, identification, and application. Mob Genet Elements 2013; 3(5): e26219.
[http://dx.doi.org/10.4161/mge.26219] [PMID: 24251069]

[34]   Blower TR, Pei XY, Short FL, *et al.* A processed noncoding RNA regulates an altruistic bacterial antiviral system. Nat Struct Mol Biol 2011; 18(2): 185-90.
[http://dx.doi.org/10.1038/nsmb.1981] [PMID: 21240270]

[35]   Masuda H, Tan Q, Awano N, Wu KP, Inouye M. YeeU enhances the bundling of cytoskeletal polymers of MreB and FtsZ, antagonizing the CbtA (YeeV) toxicity in *Escherichia coli*. Mol Microbiol 2012; 84(5): 979-89.
       [http://dx.doi.org/10.1111/j.1365-2958.2012.08068.x] [PMID: 22515815]

[36]   Margolin W. FtsZ and the division of prokaryotic cells and organelles. Nat Rev Mol Cell Biol 2005; 6(11): 862-71.
       [http://dx.doi.org/10.1038/nrm1745] [PMID: 16227976]

[37]   Tan Q, Awano N, Inouye M. YeeV is an *Escherichia coli* toxin that inhibits cell division by targeting the cytoskeleton proteins, FtsZ and MreB. Mol Microbiol 2011; 79(1): 109-18.
       [http://dx.doi.org/10.1111/j.1365-2958.2010.07433.x] [PMID: 21166897]

[38]   Schuster CF, Bertram R. Toxin-antitoxin systems are ubiquitous and versatile modulators of prokaryotic cell fate. FEMS Microbiol Lett 2013; 340(2): 73-85.
       [http://dx.doi.org/10.1111/1574-6968.12074] [PMID: 23289536]

[39]   Wang X, Lord DM, Cheng H-Y, *et al.* A new type V toxin-antitoxin system where mRNA for toxin GhoT is cleaved by antitoxin GhoS. Nat Chem Biol 2012; 8(10): 855-61.
       [http://dx.doi.org/10.1038/nchembio.1062] [PMID: 22941047]

[40]   Wang X, Lord DM, Hong SH, *et al.* Type II toxin/antitoxin MqsR/MqsA controls type V toxin/antitoxin GhoT/GhoS. Environ Microbiol 2013; 15(6): 1734-44.
       [http://dx.doi.org/10.1111/1462-2920.12063] [PMID: 23289863]

[41]   Aakre CD, Phung TN, Huang D, Laub MT. A bacterial toxin inhibits DNA replication elongation through a direct interaction with the β sliding clamp. Mol Cell 2013; 52(5): 617-28.
       [http://dx.doi.org/10.1016/j.molcel.2013.10.014] [PMID: 24239291]

[42]   Brantl S, Müller P. Toxin–antitoxin systems in *Bacillus subtilis*. Toxins (Basel) 2019; 11(5): 262.
       [http://dx.doi.org/10.3390/toxins11050262] [PMID: 31075979]

[43]   Yao NY, O'Donnell M. DNA replication: how does a sliding clamp slide? Curr Biol 2017; 27(5): R174-6.
       [http://dx.doi.org/10.1016/j.cub.2017.01.053] [PMID: 28267969]

[44]   Yang QE, Walsh TR. Toxin-antitoxin systems and their role in disseminating and maintaining antimicrobial resistance. FEMS Microbiol Rev 2017; 41(3): 343-53.
       [http://dx.doi.org/10.1093/femsre/fux006] [PMID: 28449040]

[45]   Ghafourian S, Good L, Sekawi Z, *et al.* The mazEF toxin-antitoxin system as a novel antibacterial target in Acinetobacter baumannii. Mem Inst Oswaldo Cruz 2014; 109(4): 502-5.
       [http://dx.doi.org/10.1590/0074-0276130601] [PMID: 25004148]

[46]   Hasegawa H, Suzuki E, Maeda S. Horizontal plasmid transfer by transformation in *Escherichia coli*: environmental factors and possible mechanisms. Front Microbiol 2018; 9: 2365.
       [http://dx.doi.org/10.3389/fmicb.2018.02365] [PMID: 30337917]

[47]   de la Cueva-Méndez G, Pimentel B. Gene and cell survival: lessons from prokaryotic plasmid R1. EMBO Rep 2007; 8(5): 458-64.
       [http://dx.doi.org/10.1038/sj.embor.7400957] [PMID: 17471262]

[48]   Bergstrom CT, Lipsitch M, Levin BR. Natural selection, infectious transfer and the existence conditions for bacterial plasmids. Genetics 2000; 155(4): 1505-19.
       [PMID: 10924453]

[49]   Hayes F. Toxins-antitoxins: plasmid maintenance, programmed cell death, and cell cycle arrest. Science 2003; 301(5639): 1496-9.
       [http://dx.doi.org/10.1126/science.1088157] [PMID: 12970556]

[50]   Soheili S, Ghafourian S, Sekawi Z, *et al.* The mazEF toxin-antitoxin system as an attractive target in clinical isolates of Enterococcus faecium and Enterococcus faecalis. Drug Des Devel Ther 2015; 9:

2553-61.
[PMID: 26005332]

[51]   Kang S-M, Kim D-H, Jin C, Lee B-J. A systematic overview of type II and III toxin-antitoxin systems with a focus on druggability. Toxins (Basel) 2018; 10(12): 515.
[http://dx.doi.org/10.3390/toxins10120515] [PMID: 30518070]

[52]   Peng J, Triplett LR, Schachterle JK, Sundin GW. Chromosomally encoded hok-sok toxin-antitoxin system in the fire blight pathogen Erwinia amylovora: identification and functional characterization. Appl Environ Microbiol 2019; 85(15): e00724-19.
[http://dx.doi.org/10.1128/AEM.00724-19] [PMID: 31101613]

[53]   Gupta K, Tripathi A, Sahu A, Varadarajan R. Contribution of the chromosomal ccdAB operon to bacterial drug tolerance. J Bacteriol 2017; 199(19): e00397-17.
[http://dx.doi.org/10.1128/JB.00397-17] [PMID: 28674066]

[54]   Al Marjani MF, Authman SH, Ali FS. Toxin–antitoxin systems and biofilm formation in bacteria. Rev Med Microbiol 2020; 31(2): 61-9.
[http://dx.doi.org/10.1097/MRM.0000000000000184]

[55]   Bagge N, Hentzer M, Andersen JB, Ciofu O, Givskov M, Høiby N. Dynamics and spatial distribution of β-lactamase expression in *Pseudomonas aeruginosa* biofilms. Antimicrob Agents Chemother 2004; 48(4): 1168-74.
[http://dx.doi.org/10.1128/AAC.48.4.1168-1174.2004] [PMID: 15047517]

[56]   Aspe M, Jensen L, Melegrito J, Sun M. The role of alginate and extracellular DNA in biofilm-meditated *Pseudomonas aeruginosa* gentamicin resistance. J Exp Microbiol Immunol 2012; 16: 42-8.

[57]   François B, Russell RJ, Murray JB, *et al.* Crystal structures of complexes between aminoglycosides and decoding A site oligonucleotides: role of the number of rings and positive charges in the specific binding leading to miscoding. Nucleic Acids Res 2005; 33(17): 5677-90.
[http://dx.doi.org/10.1093/nar/gki862] [PMID: 16214802]

[58]   Chiang W-C, Nilsson M, Jensen PØ, *et al.* Extracellular DNA shields against aminoglycosides in *Pseudomonas aeruginosa* biofilms. Antimicrob Agents Chemother 2013; 57(5): 2352-61.
[http://dx.doi.org/10.1128/AAC.00001-13] [PMID: 23478967]

[59]   Walters MC III, Roe F, Bugnicourt A, Franklin MJ, Stewart PS. Contributions of antibiotic penetration, oxygen limitation, and low metabolic activity to tolerance of *Pseudomonas aeruginosa* biofilms to ciprofloxacin and tobramycin. Antimicrob Agents Chemother 2003; 47(1): 317-23.
[http://dx.doi.org/10.1128/AAC.47.1.317-323.2003] [PMID: 12499208]

[60]   Keren I, Wu Y, Inocencio J, Mulcahy LR, Lewis K. Killing by bactericidal antibiotics does not depend on reactive oxygen species. Science 2013; 339(6124): 1213-6.
[http://dx.doi.org/10.1126/science.1232688] [PMID: 23471410]

[61]   Stewart PS. Mechanisms of antibiotic resistance in bacterial biofilms. Int J Med Microbiol 2002; 292(2): 107-13.
[http://dx.doi.org/10.1078/1438-4221-00196] [PMID: 12195733]

[62]   Sun C, Guo Y, Tang K, *et al.* MqsR/MqsA toxin/antitoxin system regulates persistence and biofilm formation in Pseudomonas putida KT2440. Front Microbiol 2017; 8: 840.
[http://dx.doi.org/10.3389/fmicb.2017.00840] [PMID: 28536573]

[63]   Ma D, Mandell JB, Donegan NP, *et al.* The toxin-antitoxin MazEF drives *Staphylococcus aureus* biofilm formation, antibiotic tolerance, and chronic infection. MBio 2019; 10(6): e01658-19.
[http://dx.doi.org/10.1128/mBio.01658-19] [PMID: 31772059]

[64]   Wang Y, Wang H, Hay AJ, Zhong Z, Zhu J, Kan B. Functional RelBE-family toxin-antitoxin pairs affect biofilm maturation and intestine colonization in *Vibrio cholerae*. PLoS One 2015; 10(8): e0135696.
[http://dx.doi.org/10.1371/journal.pone.0135696] [PMID: 26275048]

[65]   Sperandio V, Torres AG, Kaper JB. Quorum sensing *Escherichia coli* regulators B and C (QseBC): a novel two-component regulatory system involved in the regulation of flagella and motility by quorum sensing in *E. coli*. Mol Microbiol 2002; 43(3): 809-21.
[http://dx.doi.org/10.1046/j.1365-2958.2002.02803.x] [PMID: 11929534]

[66]   Wood TK. Insights on *Escherichia coli* biofilm formation and inhibition from whole-transcriptome profiling. Environ Microbiol 2009; 11(1): 1-15.
[http://dx.doi.org/10.1111/j.1462-2920.2008.01768.x] [PMID: 19125816]

[67]   Patrick JE, Kearns DB. Swarming motility and the control of master regulators of flagellar biosynthesis. Mol Microbiol 2012; 83(1): 14-23.
[http://dx.doi.org/10.1111/j.1365-2958.2011.07917.x] [PMID: 22092493]

[68]   Clarke MB, Sperandio V. Transcriptional regulation of flhDC by QseBC and sigma (FliA) in enterohaemorrhagic *Escherichia coli*. Mol Microbiol 2005; 57(6): 1734-49.
[http://dx.doi.org/10.1111/j.1365-2958.2005.04792.x] [PMID: 16135237]

[69]   Kim Y, Wang X, Zhang XS, *et al. Escherichia coli* toxin/antitoxin pair MqsR/MqsA regulate toxin CspD. Environ Microbiol 2010; 12(5): 1105-21.
[http://dx.doi.org/10.1111/j.1462-2920.2009.02147.x] [PMID: 20105222]

[70]   González Barrios AF, Zuo R, Hashimoto Y, Yang L, Bentley WE, Wood TK. Autoinducer 2 controls biofilm formation in *Escherichia coli* through a novel motility quorum-sensing regulator (MqsR, B3022). J Bacteriol 2006; 188(1): 305-16.
[http://dx.doi.org/10.1128/JB.188.1.305-316.2006] [PMID: 16352847]

[71]   Blair DF, Berg HC. The MotA protein of *E. coli* is a proton-conducting component of the flagellar motor. Cell 1990; 60(3): 439-49.
[http://dx.doi.org/10.1016/0092-8674(90)90595-6] [PMID: 2154333]

[72]   Wood TK, Knabel SJ, Kwan BW. Bacterial persister cell formation and dormancy. Appl Environ Microbiol 2013; 79(23): 7116-21.
[http://dx.doi.org/10.1128/AEM.02636-13] [PMID: 24038684]

[73]   Mulcahy LR, Burns JL, Lory S, Lewis K. Emergence of *Pseudomonas aeruginosa* strains producing high levels of persister cells in patients with cystic fibrosis. J Bacteriol 2010; 192(23): 6191-9.
[http://dx.doi.org/10.1128/JB.01651-09] [PMID: 20935098]

[74]   Paul P, Sahu BR, Suar M. Plausible role of bacterial toxin-antitoxin system in persister cell formation and elimination. Mol Oral Microbiol 2019; 34(3): 97-107.
[http://dx.doi.org/10.1111/omi.12258] [PMID: 30891951]

[75]   Fisher RA, Gollan B, Helaine S. Persistent bacterial infections and persister cells. Nat Rev Microbiol 2017; 15(8): 453-64.
[http://dx.doi.org/10.1038/nrmicro.2017.42] [PMID: 28529326]

[76]   Keren I, Shah D, Spoering A, Kaldalu N, Lewis K. Specialized persister cells and the mechanism of multidrug tolerance in *Escherichia coli*. J Bacteriol 2004; 186(24): 8172-80.
[http://dx.doi.org/10.1128/JB.186.24.8172-8180.2004] [PMID: 15576765]

[77]   Do DC. The Role of Bacterial Biofilms in Chronic Infections. UC Riverside 2014.

[78]   Lewis K. Persister cells and the riddle of biofilm survival. Biochemistry (Mosc) 2005; 70(2): 267-74.
[http://dx.doi.org/10.1007/s10541-005-0111-6] [PMID: 15807669]

[79]   Guttenplan SB, Kearns DB. Regulation of flagellar motility during biofilm formation. FEMS Microbiol Rev 2013; 37(6): 849-71.
[http://dx.doi.org/10.1111/1574-6976.12018] [PMID: 23480406]

[80]   Soo VW, Wood TK. Antitoxin MqsA represses curli formation through the master biofilm regulator CsgD. Sci Rep 2013; 3: 3186.
[http://dx.doi.org/10.1038/srep03186] [PMID: 24212724]

[81]   Wang X, Kim Y, Hong SH, *et al.* Antitoxin MqsA helps mediate the bacterial general stress response. Nat Chem Biol 2011; 7(6): 359-66.
[http://dx.doi.org/10.1038/nchembio.560] [PMID: 21516113]

[82]   Ramisetty BCM, Natarajan B, Santhosh RS. mazEF-mediated programmed cell death in bacteria: "what is this?". Crit Rev Microbiol 2015; 41(1): 89-100.
[http://dx.doi.org/10.3109/1040841X.2013.804030] [PMID: 23799870]

[83]   Wen Y, Behiels E, Devreese B. Toxin-Antitoxin systems: their role in persistence, biofilm formation, and pathogenicity. Pathog Dis 2014; 70(3): 240-9.
[http://dx.doi.org/10.1111/2049-632X.12145] [PMID: 24478112]

[84]   Kohanski MA, Dwyer DJ, Hayete B, Lawrence CA, Collins JJ. A common mechanism of cellular death induced by bactericidal antibiotics. Cell 2007; 130(5): 797-810.
[http://dx.doi.org/10.1016/j.cell.2007.06.049] [PMID: 17803904]

[85]   Shah D, Zhang Z, Khodursky A, Kaldalu N, Kurg K, Lewis K. Persisters: a distinct physiological state of *E. coli*. BMC Microbiol 2006; 6(1): 53.
[http://dx.doi.org/10.1186/1471-2180-6-53] [PMID: 16768798]

[86]   Dörr T, Vulić M, Lewis K. Ciprofloxacin causes persister formation by inducing the TisB toxin in *Escherichia coli*. PLoS Biol 2010; 8(2): e1000317.
[http://dx.doi.org/10.1371/journal.pbio.1000317] [PMID: 20186264]

[87]   Morgan-Linnell SK, Hiasa H, Zechiedrich L, Nitiss JL. Assessing sensitivity to antibacterial topoisomerase II inhibitors. Current Protocols in Pharmacology 2007; 39(1): 1-3.
[http://dx.doi.org/10.1002/0471141755.ph0313s39]

[88]   Simmons LA, Foti JJ, Cohen SE, Walker GC. The SOS regulatory network 2008.
[http://dx.doi.org/10.1128/ecosalplus.5.4.3]

[89]   Singletary LA, Gibson JL, Tanner EJ, *et al.* An SOS-regulated type 2 toxin-antitoxin system. J Bacteriol 2009; 191(24): 7456-65.
[http://dx.doi.org/10.1128/JB.00963-09] [PMID: 19837801]

[90]   Vogel J, Argaman L, Wagner EGH, Altuvia S. The small RNA IstR inhibits synthesis of an SOS-induced toxic peptide. Curr Biol 2004; 14(24): 2271-6.
[http://dx.doi.org/10.1016/j.cub.2004.12.003] [PMID: 15620655]

[91]   Qin T-T, Kang H-Q, Ma P, Li P-P, Huang L-Y, Gu B. SOS response and its regulation on the fluoroquinolone resistance. Ann Transl Med 2015; 3(22): 358.
[PMID: 26807413]

[92]   Völzing KG, Brynildsen MP. Stationary-phase persisters to ofloxacin sustain DNA damage and require repair systems only during recovery. MBio 2015; 6(5): e00731-15.
[http://dx.doi.org/10.1128/mBio.00731-15] [PMID: 26330511]

[93]   Engelberg-Kulka H, Hazan R, Amitai S. mazEF: a chromosomal toxin-antitoxin module that triggers programmed cell death in bacteria. J Cell Sci 2005; 118(Pt 19): 4327-32.
[http://dx.doi.org/10.1242/jcs.02619] [PMID: 16179604]

[94]   Faridani OR, Nikravesh A, Pandey DP, Gerdes K, Good L. Competitive inhibition of natural antisense Sok-RNA interactions activates Hok-mediated cell killing in *Escherichia coli*. Nucleic Acids Res 2006; 34(20): 5915-22.
[http://dx.doi.org/10.1093/nar/gkl750] [PMID: 17065468]

[95]   Fedorec AJ, Ozdemir T, Doshi A, Rosa L, Velazquez O, Danino T, *et al.* Two new plasmid post-segregational killing mechanisms for the implementation of synthetic gene networks in *E. coli*. bioRxiv 2018; 350744.

[96]   Chopin M-C, Chopin A, Roux C. Definition of bacteriophage groups according to their lytic action on mesophilic lactic streptococci. Appl Environ Microbiol 1976; 32(6): 741-6.

[http://dx.doi.org/10.1128/AEM.32.6.741-746.1976] [PMID: 16345180]

[97]   Oechslin F. Resistance development to bacteriophages occurring during bacteriophage therapy. Viruses 2018; 10(7): 351.
[http://dx.doi.org/10.3390/v10070351] [PMID: 29966329]

[98]   Stern A, Sorek R. The phage-host arms race: shaping the evolution of microbes. BioEssays 2011; 33(1): 43-51.
[http://dx.doi.org/10.1002/bies.201000071] [PMID: 20979102]

[99]   Seed KD. Battling phages: how bacteria defend against viral attack. PLoS Pathog 2015; 11(6): e1004847.
[http://dx.doi.org/10.1371/journal.ppat.1004847] [PMID: 26066799]

[100]   Dy RL, Przybilski R, Semeijn K, Salmond GP, Fineran PC. A widespread bacteriophage abortive infection system functions through a Type IV toxin-antitoxin mechanism. Nucleic Acids Res 2014; 42(7): 4590-605.
[http://dx.doi.org/10.1093/nar/gkt1419] [PMID: 24465005]

[101]   Short FL, Akusobi C, Broadhurst WR, Salmond GPC. The bacterial Type III toxin-antitoxin system, ToxIN, is a dynamic protein-RNA complex with stability-dependent antiviral abortive infection activity. Sci Rep 2018; 8(1): 1013.
[http://dx.doi.org/10.1038/s41598-017-18696-x] [PMID: 29343718]

CHAPTER 9

Acquaintance with the Known Toxin-Antitoxin Systems in *P. aeruginosa*

M. Mahmoudi[1], **S. Ghafourian**[1,*], **A. Maleki**[2] and **B. Badakhsh**[3]

[1] *Department of Microbiology, Faculty of Medicine, Ilam University of Medical Sciences, Ilam, Iran*

[2] *Clinical Microbiology Research Center, Ilam University of Medical Sciences, Ilam, Iran*

[3] *Department of Gastroenterology, Faculty of Medicine, Ilam University of Medical Sciences, Ilam, Iran*

Abstract: Toxin-antitoxin systems have been identified in most bacteria and archaea that preservation of bacterial or archaeal population is their ultimate goal. Indeed, they are regulatory systems, which play an important role in bacterial pathogenesis as well as regular physiological processes. Although they have been assigned many vital roles (antibiotic resistance, biofilm formation, persister cell formation, plasmid maintenance, post segregational killing), their role in each bacterial species is unique. Among bacterial pathogens, *P. aeruginosa* is of great importance due to its high pathogenicity. Here, we described the most known toxin-antitoxin systems and their roles in the pathogenesis of *P. aeruginosa*. Although bioinformatics studies have presented a large number of them, we have described those TA systems that have been confirmed by molecular tests. Acquaintance to TA systems and their role in *P. aeruginosa* will help to find novel ways of treatment.

Keywords: HicAB, HigBA, ParDE, RelBE.

Many TA systems have been identified in *P. aeruginosa* that have been linked to the severity of its pathogenesis. Various methods have been used to identify TA systems and the results of all of them are valuable. Many of the available data are the results of bioinformatics analysis, which predicts the status of TAs in *P. aeruginosa* as well as many other microorganisms. RASTA-Bacteria is one of the best available databases that provides TAs identification in prokaryotes (http://genoweb1.irisa.fr/duals/RASTA-Bacteria/) [1]. Subsequently, Molecular methods have higher accuracy and precision. So, PCR-based techniques are widely used to identify and investigate their features. Here, we have tried to

---

[*] **Corresponding author S. Ghafourian:** Department of Microbiology, Faculty of Medicine, Ilam University of Medical Sciences, Iran; E-mail: sobhan.ghafurian@gmail.com

introduce the main TA systems that have been molecularly confirmed in *P. aeruginosa*. Besides, their responsibility and features also have been discussed. It should be noted that the data about the specific TA system in the specific microorganism is very rare. Therefore, scientists are still trying to discover them. In the following, major TAs systems are the main topics of the discussion.

1. HIGBA TA SYSTEM

HigBA TA system belongs to the type II and consists of antitoxin HigA and toxin HigB. It is one of the main TA systems that can be found in several bacterial pathogens. In this regard, several studies indicated that it can be found abundantly on the chromosome of *P. aeruginosa* [2]. Commonly, the antitoxin gene located upstream of the toxin gene [3]. But HigB/HigA has a reverse arrangement, which means the toxin gene *higB* located at the upstream of the antitoxin gene *higA*. In addition, there are other TA systems with the reverse arrangement of genes including *mqsRA*, *hicAB*, and *brnTA* [4].

HigB/HigA considered as bona fide TA system, which means it mostly suppresses some pathogenic factors. However, inductive properties have also been reported. In this way, active HigB causes repression of pyochelin, swarming, and biofilm formation while it causes induction of type three secretion system (T3SS) [5, 6]. HigA controls the activity of HigB through different ways, which we will explain further.

In the logarithmic phase of growth, HigA and HigB are produced in equal amounts. Therefore, HigB neutralized by HigA inside the bacterial cell. But in late stationary phase of growth, HigA produced more than HigB. The excess HigA biding to its own promotor region named *mvfR* and repressed the transcription of the operon. Therefore, the genes under the control of *mvfR* promoter are suppressed. The extra *higA* mRNA expressed from the other promotor, which is located inside of the *higB* region. As a result, by the suppression of the *higB*, pyochelin production, biofilm formation, and swarming will be increased. But there is another interesting point here. LasR, a quorum-sensing regulator, controls the production of pyocyanin. The translational site of *mvfR* is located downstream of the *lasR* binding site. Also, the binding site of the higA in the mvfR promotor is located downstream of the *lasR* binding site. This very close proximity between components of quorum-sensing and TA loci creates complexities. In the simple words, the high level of HigA can inactivate HigB, which leads to the production of swarming, biofilm formation and pyochelin. Subsequently, extra HigA can disrupts the production of pyocyanin by impressing the LasR [7].

As was mentioned, one of the features of TA systems is the survival of the bacterial cell under the stress condition. For example, nutrient, pH and heat stress, antibiotics, immune response, *etc.* these factors can activate cellular proteases like Lon protease [8]. As the antitoxin HigA is labile, it can be degraded by Lon protease.

Therefore, HigB can repress the production of pyochelin, biofilm formation, and motility. On the other hand, there is no extra HigA to disrupt the production of pyocyanin. So the pyocyanin will be produced under the stress condition along with HigB (Fig. **1**) [7].

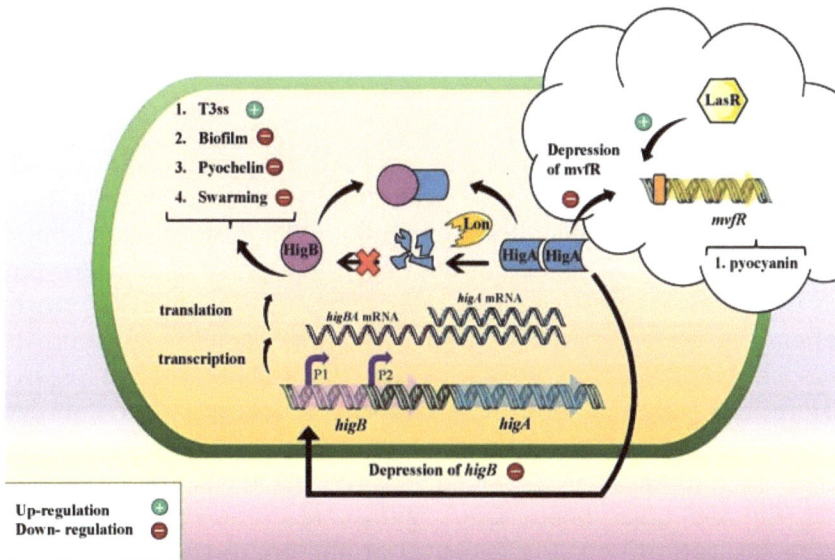

Fig. (1). The effect of HigB on virulence factors of *P. aeruginosa*. HigA and HigB are expressed in different terms with different values. In detail, HigA and HigB are evenly expressed in the exponential phase of growth while HigA is expressed to a greater extent in the late stationary phase of growth. By the more production of HigA, *mvfR* and the genes it controls will be suppressed. Besides, HigA could be degraded by Lon protease under the special conditions, which results in suppression of *higB* and *mvfR*. HigB down-regulates biofilm formation, production of pyochelin, and swarming while it up-regulates the production of T3SS. When HigA binds to the HigB, HigA inhibits the HigB toxicity through neutralization. In addition, the HigA-HigB complex causes a reduction in binding of HigA to the promotor of *mvfR* or *higB*.

Besides, HigA/HigB has been identified in other important pathogens including, *E. coli* O157:H7, *E. coli* K12, *E. coli* CFT073, *Mycobacterium tuberculosis*, *Acinetobacter baumannii*, *Yersinia pestis*, *Vibrio cholera*, *Streptococcus pneumonia*, *etc.* [5].

2. HICAB TA SYSTEM

HicAB belongs to type II TA systems that HicA and HicB are the toxin and antitoxin, respectively [9]. One of the features of HicAB TA system is that HicA protein is larger than HicB protein [10]. In addition, *P. aeruginosa* obtained *hisAB* by horizontal gene transfer. So it is located on plasmid or part of the prophage genomes. In the normal condition, *hicA* and *hicB* transcribed together through bicistronic operon. In 2016, Gang Li *et al.*, identified the HicAB TA system in *P. aeruginosa*. Besides, they demonstrated that HicAB is not involved in biofilm formation and virulence. But the HicAB is located at the conserved region of the genome, which probably means it play a key role in cellular process [9]. Unfortunately, it has not been proven yet and needs future studies.

3. PARDE TA SYSTEM

ParDE belongs to the type II TA system. ParD and ParE proteins are antitoxin and toxin, respectively. In 1990, Roberts *et al.* identified *parDE* locus on plasmid RK2. ParE toxin impeded gyrase mediated supercoiling that leads to the inhibition of cell proliferation. DNA-gyrase is one of the bacterial topoisomerase enzymes, which requires ATP to creates negative supercoils in DNA [11]. During replication, helicase enzyme separates double stranded DNA by breaking the hydrogen bonds ahead of the DNA polymerase III, which produce positive supercoiling. Here, DNA gyrase moves in front of the helicase and stabilized DNA helix by creates negative super coiling. Consequently, relaxed DNA strains will be available for polymerization, which is very crucial situation in DNA replication [12]. On the other hand, DNA gyrase has indirect role in gene expression due to susceptibility of the bacterial promotors to supercoiling [13]. Since DNA gyrase presents in all bacteria while it is absent in eukaryotic cells, it is considered as very valuable antibacterial target. In parallel, all DNA gyrase inhibitors are precious to the same extent [14].

For more clarity, here, we explained the mode of action and effect of the quinolone antibiotics, the famous DNA gyrase inhibitors, on the bacterial cell. These antibiotics arrest DNA-DNA gyrase complex and prevent religation. Therefore, this complex does not allow the replication fork to move forward and continue to DNA replication. This event leads todouble-strand break of DNA and fragmentation of bacterial chromosome. So, the bacterial cell goes to the death [15].

Interestingly, ParE toxin also targets the DNA gyrase, which will be explained in the following. In 2002, *Jiang, et al.* detected *parDE* locus on Broad-host-range plasmid RK2 as postsegregational killing system in *E. coli*. This system maintains the RK2 plasmid during the bacterial cell division. The active ParE inhibited DNA replication in both plasmid and chromosome that leads to the production of filamentous cell and bacterial death. Moreover, they also demonstrated that bacterial death is due to the inhibition of gyrase activity by ParE. While with the presence of ParD, gyrase could not be inhibited by the ParE, and bacteria will survive. Overall, this study demonstrated the toxic effect of ParE when it is located on a plasmid [16]. Nevertheless, many ParDE operons were found on the chromosome, which led scientists to explore other possible properties.

In 2019, Muthuramalingam, *et al.* demonstrated the protective role of toxin ParE to anti-gyrase antibiotics in *P. aeruginosa*. More precisely, they indicated that the effect of the ParE is concentration-dependent and vary from protective to toxic. They confirmed that *P. aeruginosa* ParE can inhibit the supercoiling activity of DNA gyrase. Also, the over expression of ParE in the absence of ParD is deadly for *P. aeruginosa*. But in the normal status, the ParE monomer interacts with ParD dimer and forms heterodimer. In consequence, they indicated that ParE can interact with DNA gyrase and inhibits its activity or protects it from the effect of other inhibitors. Each of these two conditions depends on the dose of active ParE. Unfortunately, the process of shifting between these two statuses remained unknown and needs more studies [17].

4. RELBE TA SYSTEM

RelBE consists of RelB and RelE antitoxin and toxin, respectively. The high expression of *relE* causes severe inhibition of the translation that leads to the bacterial cell destruction. Therefore, this molecule should be under the limitation of an antidote. Thus, RelB is responsible for neutralizing RelE. RelBE belongs to the type II TA system and both are proteins [18].

RelBEF operon consists of promoter (Pr), *relB*, *relE* and *relF,* respectively. *relB* and *relE* belong to the TA systems and *relF* is one of the members of Hok cytotoxin family.

After the expression of RelB and RelE, they bond together and form a monomer and then dimer. Antitoxin relB suppresses the activation of Pr to inhibit the transcription. All forms of relB, free or bounded are able to inhibit the Pr. Here, another molecule, Lon protease enters, that changes this neutral system. The Lon protease degrades antitoxin RelB, and these results in freedom of RelB toxin [19].

Now, free toxin RelBE is able to inhibit the transcription inside the bacterial cell.

For this purpose, RelE assails to the stalled ribosomes by its RNase activity. The target sites for RelE are bounded mRNAs to the ribosome. But, it can cleave mRNAs at both stop and sense codons. In detail, these stop codons are UAG > UAA > UGA and sense codons are CAG and UCG [20].

Here, tmRNA's rescue system comes to the scene. Briefly, the tmRNA rescue system is a quality control system that surveils protein production. Sometimes, some stalled translation complexes form that must be recycled. Therefore, recycling these materials is the responsibility of tmRNA ribosome-rescue system [21].

After the effects of toxin RelE, the ribosome will be blocked and the truncated mRNAs in A site will be formed. The tmRNA rescue system identifies this structure. Here, tmRNA perches on A site and accepts the nascent chain form the P site. Now the tmRNA molecule has two district special parts. One of them is the protein nascent chain and another one is the mRNA-like part (the truncated mRNAs). Eventfully, this tagged nascent chain goes for degradation and this is how protein synthesis stops (Fig. **2**) [22].

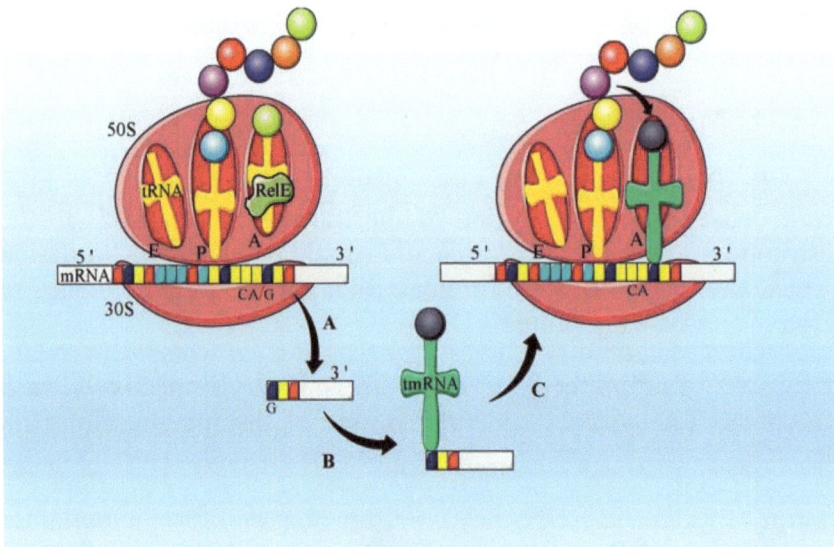

Fig. (2). The effect of the RelE on translation. In general, RelE causes inhibition of protein synthesis. Free RelE assails to stalled ribosomes by making an incision at the second position of the A site codon. In the present figure, the second position of the A site is adenosine of CAG codon of the mRNA. As a result, the ribosome is blocked and the mRNA becomes truncated. This structure is attractive for the tmRNA rescue system and plays the role of the substrate. At this time, the tmRNA molecule binds to the A site and received the nascent protein chain from lateral tRNA, which is located at the P site. The translation also continues from the truncated mRNA part of tmRNA. By this process, the nascent chain tagged and goes to degradation.

However, in 2011 Williams and coworkers reported that *relBE* was presented in 100% (n=42) of *P. aeruginosa* clinical isolates for the first time. Due to the high prevalence and properties of *relBE*, they suggested that toxin could be the potential antimicrobial target for *P. aeruginosa* [23].

This issue provided basis for future research and it drew scientists' attention to the role of RelBE in *P. aeruginosa.*

In recent years, a study also demonstrated 100% (n=92) prevalence of *relBE* that was associated with resistance to aztreonam. Obviously, they observed that the level of the expression of *relBE* gene is increased in sensitive aztreonam isolates (isolates sensitive to aztreonam) compare with those that are resistant to aztreonam. The association between expressions of *relBE* and sensitivity to aztreonam among *P. aeruginosa* isolates led to the creation of an idea. Therefore, maybe by increasing the level of relBE, the antibiotic resistance can be reduced [24].

CONSENT FOR PUBLICATION

Not applicable.

CONFLICT OF INTEREST

The authors declare no conflict of interest, financial or otherwise.

ACKNOWLEDGEMENTS

Declared none.

REFERENCES

[1]   Sevin EW, Barloy-Hubler F. RASTA-Bacteria: a web-based tool for identifying toxin-antitoxin loci in prokaryotes. Genome Biol 2007; 8(8): R155.
[http://dx.doi.org/10.1186/gb-2007-8-8-r155] [PMID: 17678530]

[2]   Savari M, Rostami S, Ekrami A, Bahador A. Characterization of toxin-antitoxin (TA) systems in *Pseudomonas aeruginosa* clinical isolates in Iran. Jundishapur J Microbiol 2016; 9(1)e26627
[http://dx.doi.org/10.5812/jjm.26627] [PMID: 27099681]

[3]   De Bruijn FJ. Stress and environmental regulation of gene expression and adaptation in bacteria. John Wiley & Sons 2016.
[http://dx.doi.org/10.1002/9781119004813]

[4]   Liu Y, Gao Z, Liu G, Geng Z, Dong Y, Zhang H. Structural insights into the transcriptional regulation of HigBA toxin-antitoxin system by antitoxin HigA in *Pseudomonas aeruginosa*. Front Microbiol 2020; 10: 3158.
[http://dx.doi.org/10.3389/fmicb.2019.03158] [PMID: 32038588]

[5]   Wood TL, Wood TK. The HigB/HigA toxin/antitoxin system of *Pseudomonas aeruginosa* influences the virulence factors pyochelin, pyocyanin, and biofilm formation. MicrobiologyOpen 2016; 5(3): 499-511.

[http://dx.doi.org/10.1002/mbo3.346] [PMID: 26987441]

[6]   Zhang Y, Xia B, Li M, *et al.* HigB reciprocally controls biofilm formation and the expression of type III secretion system genes through influencing the intracellular c-di-GMP level in *Pseudomonas aeruginosa.* Toxins (Basel) 2018; 10(11): 424.
[http://dx.doi.org/10.3390/toxins10110424] [PMID: 30355991]

[7]   Guo Y, Sun C, Li Y, Tang K, Ni S, Wang X. Antitoxin HigA inhibits virulence gene mvfR expression in *Pseudomonas aeruginosa.* Environ Microbiol 2019; 21(8): 2707-23.
[http://dx.doi.org/10.1111/1462-2920.14595] [PMID: 30882983]

[8]   Coussens NP, Daines DA. Wake me when it's over - Bacterial toxin-antitoxin proteins and induced dormancy. Exp Biol Med (Maywood) 2016; 241(12): 1332-42.
[http://dx.doi.org/10.1177/1535370216651938] [PMID: 27216598]

[9]   Li G, Shen M, Lu S, *et al.* Identification and characterization of the HicAB toxin-antitoxin system in the opportunistic pathogen *Pseudomonas aeruginosa.* Toxins (Basel) 2016; 8(4): 113.
[http://dx.doi.org/10.3390/toxins8040113] [PMID: 27104566]

[10]   Jørgensen MG, Pandey DP, Jaskolska M, Gerdes K. HicA of *Escherichia coli* defines a novel family of translation-independent mRNA interferases in bacteria and archaea. J Bacteriol 2009; 191(4): 1191-9.
[http://dx.doi.org/10.1128/JB.01013-08] [PMID: 19060138]

[11]   Roberts RC, Burioni R, Helinski DR. Genetic characterization of the stabilizing functions of a region of broad-host-range plasmid RK2. J Bacteriol 1990; 172(11): 6204-16.
[http://dx.doi.org/10.1128/JB.172.11.6204-6216.1990] [PMID: 2121707]

[12]   Ashley RE, Dittmore A, McPherson SA, Turnbough CL Jr, Neuman KC, Osheroff N. Activities of gyrase and topoisomerase IV on positively supercoiled DNA. Nucleic Acids Res 2017; 45(16): 9611-24.
[http://dx.doi.org/10.1093/nar/gkx649] [PMID: 28934496]

[13]   Travers A, Muskhelishvili G. DNA supercoiling - a global transcriptional regulator for enterobacterial growth? Nat Rev Microbiol 2005; 3(2): 157-69.
[http://dx.doi.org/10.1038/nrmicro1088] [PMID: 15685225]

[14]   Collin F, Karkare S, Maxwell A. Exploiting bacterial DNA gyrase as a drug target: current state and perspectives. Appl Microbiol Biotechnol 2011; 92(3): 479-97.
[http://dx.doi.org/10.1007/s00253-011-3557-z] [PMID: 21904817]

[15]   Mustaev A, Malik M, Zhao X, *et al.* Fluoroquinolone-gyrase-DNA complexes: two modes of drug binding. J Biol Chem 2014; 289(18): 12300-12.
[http://dx.doi.org/10.1074/jbc.M113.529164] [PMID: 24497635]

[16]   Jiang Y, Pogliano J, Helinski DR, Konieczny I. ParE toxin encoded by the broad-host-range plasmid RK2 is an inhibitor of *Escherichia coli* gyrase. Mol Microbiol 2002; 44(4): 971-9.
[http://dx.doi.org/10.1046/j.1365-2958.2002.02921.x] [PMID: 12010492]

[17]   Muthuramalingam M, White JC, Murphy T, Ames JR, Bourne CR. The toxin from a ParDE toxin-antitoxin system found in *Pseudomonas aeruginosa* offers protection to cells challenged with anti-gyrase antibiotics. Mol Microbiol 2019; 111(2): 441-54.
[http://dx.doi.org/10.1111/mmi.14165] [PMID: 30427086]

[18]   Christensen SK, Gerdes K. RelE toxins from bacteria and Archaea cleave mRNAs on translating ribosomes, which are rescued by tmRNA. Mol Microbiol 2003; 48(5): 1389-400.
[http://dx.doi.org/10.1046/j.1365-2958.2003.03512.x] [PMID: 12787364]

[19]   Yamamoto T-A, Gerdes K, Tunnacliffe A. Bacterial toxin RelE induces apoptosis in human cells. FEBS Lett 2002; 519(1-3): 191-4.
[http://dx.doi.org/10.1016/S0014-5793(02)02764-3] [PMID: 12023043]

[20]   Takagi H, Kakuta Y, Okada T, Yao M, Tanaka I, Kimura M. Crystal structure of archaeal toxin-

antitoxin RelE-RelB complex with implications for toxin activity and antitoxin effects. Nat Struct Mol Biol 2005; 12(4): 327-31.
[http://dx.doi.org/10.1038/nsmb911] [PMID: 15768033]

[21]   Janssen BD, Hayes CS. The tmRNA ribosome-rescue system Advances in protein chemistry and structural biology 86. Elsevier 2012; pp. 151-91.

[22]   Wilson DN, Nierhaus KH. RelBE or not to be. Nat Struct Mol Biol 2005; 12(4): 282-4.
[http://dx.doi.org/10.1038/nsmb0405-282] [PMID: 15809644]

[23]   Williams JJ, Halvorsen EM, Dwyer EM, DiFazio RM, Hergenrother PJ. Toxin-antitoxin (TA) systems are prevalent and transcribed in clinical isolates of *Pseudomonas aeruginosa* and methicillin-resistant *Staphylococcus* aureus. FEMS Microbiol Lett 2011; 322(1): 41-50.
[http://dx.doi.org/10.1111/j.1574-6968.2011.02330.x] [PMID: 21658105]

[24]   Coskun USS, Cicek AC, Kilinc C, *et al.* Effect of mazEF, higBA and relBE toxin-antitoxin systems on antibiotic resistance in *Pseudomonas aeruginosa* and *Staphylococcus* isolates. Malawi Med J 2018; 30(2): 67-72.
[http://dx.doi.org/10.4314/mmj.v30i2.3] [PMID: 30627331]

SUBJECT INDEX

A

Absorption 12, 82
  high 12
  preventing 82
Acid 10, 13, 16, 23, 62, 82
  arachidonic 23
  β-D-mannuronic 13
  clavulanic 62
  Ethylenediaminetetraacetic 10
  nucleic 82
  phenazine a-carboxylic 16
Acidic vesicular organelles 15
Acinetobacter baumannii 70, 93
Acinetobacter spp 39
Acquired immunity 11
Activity 12, 16, 19, 20, 22, 24, 25, 46, 63, 69,
    71, 72, 73, 74, 82, 83, 92, 95
  antibacterial 16
  antimicrobial 24
  antiphage 82, 83
  elastic metalloproteinase 25
  endoribonuclease 74
  enzymatic 20, 69
  histidine kinase 19
  interferase 71
  intermediate nephrotoxic 63
  tyrosine-kinase 25
Acyl-homoserine lactones (AHLs) 18
Addiction, morphine 46
Adhesion site 13
ADP-ribosylation 22
  activity 22
  reaction 22
ADP-ribosyltransferase activity 22
Adrenocortical cells 21
Alginate 8, 9, 13, 17, 19, 76
  and eDNA sequester 76
  producer bacteria 13
Amino acid 22, 78
  deficiency 78
  homology 22

Aminoglycosides 10, 49, 59, 60, 63, 76
  semisynthetic 63
Antibacterial effect 16
Antibiotic resistance 17, 59, 60, 61, 62, 63,
    68, 69, 70, 74, 75, 76, 77, 91
  genes 59, 60, 61, 75
  intrinsic 60
  mechanisms of 61, 76
  severe 59, 61
  systems influence 75
  treatment 61, 63
Antibiotic(s) 13, 48, 49, 59, 60, 61, 62, 63, 75,
    76, 78, 79, 94, 95
  anti-gyrase 95
  beta-lactam 61, 62
  carbapenem 63
  combat 60
  novel 62
  quinolone 94
  transport 61
    susceptibility 63
    therapy condition 13
Antitoxin 68, 69, 70, 71, 72, 73, 74, 75, 77,
    78, 80, 81, 83, 92
  encode 69
  gene 92
  molecules 75
  unstable 81
Astrocytoma cells 15
Atelectasis 23
Athlete's foot infection 48
Aztreonam 62, 63, 97
  sensitive 97

B

Bacillus 5, 6, 16, 24, 39
  aeruginosus 6
  anthracis 16
  cereus 39
  pyocyaneus 5, 6
  subtilis 24

www.ingramcontent.com/pod-product-compliance
Lightning Source LLC
Chambersburg PA
CBHW041718210326
41598CB00007B/702